"Elyse Resch packs over thirty-six years of counseling wisdom and intuitive eating expertise into this welcome resource for teens, which will help them overcome the bondage of diet culture and body dissatisfaction. *The Intuitive Eating Workbook for Teens* is chock-full of tips and helpful exercises, and written in a way that teens will easily connect with, such as how to deal with food when it is the 'frenemy.' Health professionals will appreciate the eighty-four activities that can help their adolescent clients reconnect with (and trust) their own innate body wisdom."

—**Evelyn Tribole, MS, RDN, CEDRD-S**, is coauthor of *Intuitive Eating* and *The Intuitive Eating Workbook*, and has a private counseling practice in Newport Beach, CA

"Many years ago, when I gave up dieting for intuitive eating, I felt relief! I was no longer obsessed with food or disliked my body. Intuitive eating continues to enhance my well-being. *The Intuitive Eating Workbook for Teens* will do this for you. Elyse Resch is the world's leading authority on intuitive eating, and her ideas on intuitive eating are confirmed by hundreds of research studies. In this workbook, she has distilled the ten principles of intuitive eating into many thought-provoking and effective activities that will help all teens make peace with food and their bodies."

—**Tracy Tylka, PhD**, professor, editor-in-chief of *Body Image*, and coeditor of *Handbook of Positive Body Image and Embodiment*

"Having overcome my own eating disorder (that began in my teens), and having spent the last several decades helping teens in my psychotherapy practice, I know the immense benefits that the intuitive eating process can offer to a young person's life. Elyse lays it all out beautifully in this important workbook. The original *Intuitive Eating* book introduced us to a life-changing concept. This teen version will do nothing less."

—**Andrea Wachter, LMFT**, author of *Getting Over Overeating for Teens*, and coauthor of *Mirror, Mirror on the Wall* and *The Don't Diet, Live-It Workbook*

"Brilliant, best-selling author and dietitian Elyse Resch has done it again with this wonderful workbook designed to help teenagers learn how to eat in a balanced, joyful, intuitive way. This fun, interactive, and comprehensive guide encourages teens to consider how the toxic effects of social media and harmful 'diet culture' messages—as well as their own sense of self-confidence and emotional states—affect their relationship with food and their bodies. In honoring body diversity and bringing commonsense wisdom to teens, this workbook also offers highly medically sound advice. I will definitely be recommending it for my teenage patients!"

—**Jennifer L. Gaudiani, MD, CEDS, FAED**, founder and medical director, Gaudiani Clinic

"I wish I'd had *The Intuitive Eating Workbook for Teens* by Elyse Resch when I was a teenager to teach me the dangers of chronic dieting and how to identify hunger, cravings, satisfaction, and fullness. This workbook covers all this and more—how to stop making comparisons with others, value your body, shower yourself with compassion, and assign food a healthy place in your life. Resch's expertise in feeding ourselves shines through on every page and makes the workbook a perfect read for adolescents hungry for knowledge about how to eat well and take care of their bodies."

—**Karen R. Koenig, LCSW, Med**, is an eating psychology expert, popular blogger, and author of seven books on eating, weight, and body image, including *Outsmarting Overeating* and *The Rules of "Normal" Eating*

"I love this workbook! I work with adult survivors of childhood abuse, and that abuse has interfered with their ability to take care of themselves and to develop a healthy relationship with food and their bodies. For teens who read and use this workbook, they will be given the tools to learn to trust their inner voice in ways that my clients have not. Their relationship with food and their bodies is fundamental to creating a happy and healthy life. I wish my clients had had this workbook when they were teens."

—**Arlene Drake, PhD, LMFT**, is a psychotherapist who is an expert in treating adult survivors of childhood abuse, and is author of *Carefrontation*

"Elyse Resch has done it again with this must-have, go-to guide for teens, their parents, and treatment professionals! The principles of intuitive eating come to life in new ways with practical activities and relatable examples through Elyse's compassionate, non-parental tone. This book will prevent teens from dieting and disordered eating, offering them a clear path to a relationship with food and themselves during the teen years and beyond. This book offers endless wisdom and actionable steps that anyone can use. I can't recommend this book highly enough!"

—**Janean Anderson, PhD, CEDS-S**, licensed psychologist, certified eating disorders specialist, host, The Eating Disorder Recovery Podcast, best-selling author of *Recover Your Perspective*, founder and director, Colorado Therapy & Assessment Center

"Social media, consumer culture, and high school health class surround our kids in a sea of nutrition misinformation without a raft. Enter *The Intuitive Eating Workbook for Teens*—a lifesaver crafted of IE wisdom, encouragement to rebel against diet rules, and worksheets that tap into personal truths. Until every teen has a personal dietitian, they should all get a copy of this book."

—**Jessica Setnick, MS, RD, CEDRD-S**, director of The International Federation of Eating Disorder Dietitians, and author of *The Eating Disorders Clinical Pocket Guide*

"Intuitive eating changed my life. I only wish I'd known about these transformative principles when I was a teen. Read this book to make peace with food and your body!"

—**Jenni Schaefer**, author of *Life Without Ed*; *Almost Anorexic*; and *Goodbye Ed, Hello Me*

"This is the book we've been waiting for! In *The Intuitive Eating Workbook for Teens*, Resch compassionately offers her fresh perspective on eating for teens who don't want to diet. I would recommend a copy for everyone, as it provides smart guidance and empowers teen readers to let go of stress with food and body using the proven science of intuitive eating."

—**Sumner Brooks, MPH, RDN, CEDRD**, is an eating disorder dietitian, creator of EDRD Pro for eating disorder professionals, and coauthor of *Savvy Girl*

"As diet culture continues to influence younger and younger populations, eating disorders continue to rise exponentially. Elyse unmasks the veil of diet culture, blasts through society and cultural standards, and speaks with kindness and compassion to our world's youth. Despite the serious, challenging nature of the workbook, Elyse speaks with a 'cool factor' that particularly resonates with youth and teens everywhere. *The Intuitive Eating Workbook for Teens* is a true godsend to teens everywhere, no matter your culture or socioeconomic status!"

—**Stefani Reinold, MD, MPH**, board-certified psychiatrist, author of *Let Your Heart Out*, and host of the podcast *It's Not About the Food*

"*The Intuitive Eating Workbook for Teens* is a vital resource that is sure to help teens everywhere create a healthier relationship with food. How wonderful that this foundation of health be built early, while the brain is still developing, and the habit of self-care can be instilled, lasting a lifetime. It is comprehensive, interactive, and well written. This is a must-have read for teens!"

—**Maryann Jacobsen, MS, RD**, author of *How to Raise a Mindful Eater*, and coauthor of *Fearless Feeding*

"*Intuitive Eating* changed my life, and I only wish I had found it when I was a teenager. It would have saved me so much anguish and given me back the many years I spent in the cycle of dieting, disordered eating, and self-loathing. I can think of no better—or more important—gift to bestow upon a young person struggling with food and body image. It is a guiding light through the chaos of diet culture, encouraging an unshakeable self-respect and commonsense approach to food, fitness, and body acceptance."

—**Kelsey Miller**, creator of The Anti-Diet Project, and author of *Big Girl* and *I'll Be There for You*

"With clarity and kindness, *The Intuitive Eating Workbook for Teens* offers a reliable structure for healing your relationship to food and learning to trust your body. I wish I had this book when I was a dieting teen! It would have made all the difference when I was feeling vulnerable to weight and body concerns."

—**Rebecca Scritchfield, RDN, EP-C**, author of *Body Kindness*

"I will be recommending *The Intuitive Eating Workbook for Teens* far and wide! In today's diet culture, teens are constantly exposed to messages about food, dieting, and weight that often result in eating struggles and poor body image. Through easy-to-understand information and engaging activities, Elyse Resch offers an invaluable resource to help teens develop a lifelong positive and nourishing relationship with food and their bodies. Parents will also benefit from reading this workbook so that they can fully support their teens in letting go of the diet mentality and becoming intuitive eaters. Thank you, Elyse!"

—**Judith Matz**, coauthor of *The Diet Survivor's Handbook* and *Beyond a Shadow of a Diet*

the intuitive eating workbook for teens

a non-diet, body positive approach to building a healthy relationship with food

ELYSE RESCH, MS, RDN

Instant Help Books

An Imprint of New Harbinger Publications, Inc.

Distributed in Canada by Raincoast Books

Copyright © 2019 by Elyse Resch
          Instant Help Books
          An imprint of New Harbinger Publications, Inc.
          5674 Shattuck Avenue
          Oakland, CA 94609
          www.newharbinger.com

INSTANT HELP, the Clock Logo, and NEW HARBINGER are trademarks of New Harbinger Publications, Inc.

Cover design by Amy Shoup

Acquired by Ryan Buresh

Edited by Karen Schader

Illustrations by Russelle Marcato Westbrook

Library of Congress Cataloging-in-Publication Data on file

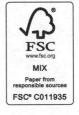
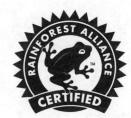

22   21   20

10   9   8   7   6   5   4   3   2

To every teen who has struggled with your relationship with food and your body—I offer you a path to the freedom and joy that comes with trusting your inner wisdom as an intuitive eater.

And to Michael Resch, my son, the original intuitive eater and love of my life.

Contents

Introduction

In some ways, I was super lucky when I was a teenager. Nobody I knew at school talked about weight or bodies. Maybe it was because I didn't hang with the kids who did. Or, maybe, people just weren't so body focused.

For you, though, it's likely that many of your friends are obsessed with something called the culturally thin ideal. We live in a world that promotes being thin as a lofty goal. Because of this, you're probably hearing a lot of body-bashing comments—people saying nasty things about the size or shape of their bodies, because they think they don't match up. Kids of all genders feel the pressure for body perfection. They talk about how they're sure life would be so much better if only they could buy clothes in a smaller size. Or you may hear them saying that they believe they'd be more popular if they had "six-packs." Essentially, all teens can be affected by an appearance-oriented world. Regardless of where they fall on the gender spectrum, many teens are victims of these unrealistic demands. They're hating their bodies and fantasizing that they'll be liked or admired more if only their bodies were "perfect."

It's not surprising that this kind of thinking is so widespread among kids. Adults often think and feel the same way. Your mother may talk about how fat she feels or how she wishes she could just not eat any carbs (as if this were a positive goal!); your father may be upset that he doesn't have the taut muscles he had in college. And even if your parents aren't talking this way, you may hear your doctor say things like, "I'm worried about your weight—you've gained too much this year." That can make you feel bad and inadequate and even scared.

You're also seeing magazine ads using photoshopped pictures of models that look perfect to you, making you feel even more inadequate, and you're bombarded by images of unrealistically thin and flawlessly muscular bodies on TV and in the movies.

And then there's social media: a constant reminder that you're not good enough. Social media celebrities—and even your friends—post pictures of themselves looking as if they have perfect lives. (Of course, people post those pictures only on their best days. And, like everyone, they've probably deleted all the ones on their phones that they think make them look bad. They would never post those!)

Instead of questioning these images or any of the conversations that are going on about this drive for beauty, thinness, and perfection, you may find yourself driven to talk about depressing, anxiety-triggering things like needing to lose weight, debating good versus bad foods, and feeling fat, just as often or even more often than you talk about things that are positive and make you feel happy, like your crushes and your favorite music.

You may believe that you're not good enough just as you are; you may have been tempted to go on diets so you can get the perfect body. But here's the thing: diets are doomed to failure and can have some serious negative side effects. Many people who diet go on to bingeing after they fall off the diet. Also, when you hear that someone is on a diet, it's a good bet that there could be a future eating disorder in the making. And what's really scary is that young kids who diet have a big chance of developing an eating disorder by the time they're in their teens.

Sounds like terrible news, right? It does *not* have to be, because there is another way. Intuitive eating, which you'll be learning about in this workbook, is about being comfortable with who you are, both inside and out, and becoming liberated from the external pressures to conform.

You'll learn what you need to fight the influences social media, TV, movies, your parents, and maybe even your doctor have on you. You'll learn to have a good, healthy relationship with your body—and with food—in spite of all the messages that make you feel that's just not possible for you.

Intuitive Eating is a philosophy based on the belief that most people are born with all the wisdom they need to know how to eat in a satisfying and balanced way. If you've lost touch with this wisdom—and so many of us have—Intuitive Eating helps you reconnect with it. It helps you become more body positive and promises you a sense of freedom to truly enjoy all foods and to feel the safety that comes with trusting your wise body.

Over ninety research studies have focused on the benefits of intuitive eating. These studies have shown that intuitive eaters have better coping skills; higher self-esteem; a greater sense of well-being; more optimism, body appreciation, and acceptance; more awareness of signals their body gives them, psychological strength, and unconditional self-regard; and, most important, more pleasure from eating. From a medical standpoint, intuitive eaters are also found to be physically healthier in many ways. So how does this all sound to you? Intriguing, I hope!

The Principles of Intuitive Eating

Intuitive Eating is made up of ten steps or principles:

- Reject the Diet Mentality. This principle teaches you about what's wrong with dieting and why you're going to want to ditch this miserable process.

- Honor Your Hunger. Here you'll learn about your personal relationship with hunger—whether you are usually hungry as a bear, ignore your hunger, or are tuned into normal hunger.

- Make Peace with Food. Find out if you're living in Food Jail, believing that there are "good" foods and "bad" foods. (Hint: there aren't.) And you'll learn to challenge all the rules about eating that have kept you imprisoned.

- Challenge the Food Police. If you find yourself in Food Jail, you might need to ask: who is keeping you imprisoned, and how do you free yourself?

- Feel Your Fullness. This principle guides you to think about whether you eat and eat until you're uncomfortable and even miserable, and helps you learn why and how to stop eating when you're comfortably full.

- Discover the Satisfaction Factor. Just how yummy are your meals? They should be deliciously satisfying. If they're not, this principle sets you on the path to more eating enjoyment.

- Cope with Your Emotions Without Using Food. Is food your best friend or your enemy? Maybe it's both. With Intuitive Eating, you'll find ways to separate your emotions from your eating.

- Respect Your Body. Is your body your temple, your fortress, or your foe? Here, you'll learn to take loving care of your one and only wonderful body.

- Exercise—Feel the Difference. Are you a couch potato or an energizer bunny? Find out how to make movement and activity a happy part of your life.

- Honor Your Health with Gentle Nutrition. From nutrition to play food—there's room for it all. It's the key to feeling healthier, happier, and guilt-free!

These principles are usually taught in the order listed above. In this book, though, the order is a bit different, because you're a bit different. I decided to teach you about the principles in the order I think will be the most helpful for you, a young person whose body and experiences are growing and changing.

How to Use This Workbook

As you read this workbook, you'll learn many new facts and will be offered activities that will help you explore this new way of thinking and change how you view food and your body.
There are three main ways to accomplish this:

1. You can do your work within the workbook itself. There are spaces after each activity for your reflections and comments on the exercises.

2. You can also use a notebook to record the thoughts that come up for you while doing the exercises. This will become the central place to hold your work. If you use a loose-leaf binder, you'll be able to insert pages for more writing over time, as well as any checklists

or charts you fill out and any drawings or pictures you'd like to add. Your notebook will become your treasure and your sacred place to return to over and over once you finish the workbook, and it will store your progress in becoming an intuitive eater. Repeated practice will help you strengthen the skills you're learning, and you'll be able to go back to your notebook to find the activities any time you need them.

3. On the New Harbinger website—http://www.newharbinger.com/41443—you'll find downloadable PDFs of some of the charts and worksheets, which you can print and use to make as many copies as you need to practice your new skills. Be sure to add them to your notebook.

This is a wonderful moment for you to learn and practice the habits and attitudes that will free you to have a happy, healthy lifelong relationship with your body and with food. I hope you enjoy this journey!

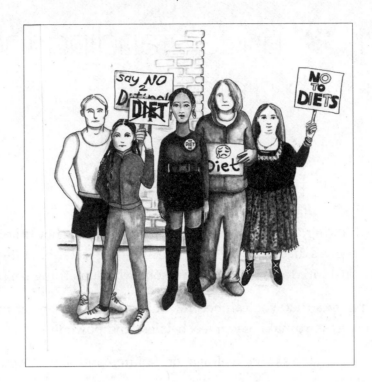

chapter 1

What's Wrong with Dieting?

You're amazingly lucky if you've never thought about going on a diet, because then you've never had that feeling of being deprived of the foods you love or being angry with yourself for not being able to stay on it. But, if you're reading this book, it's likely that you've either been on a diet, thought you should be on one, or know people who have been on diets.

> *Brooke started dieting when she was thirteen. At first she was super excited—she believed the diet would help her lose weight, and then her problems would all be solved. Unfortunately, it didn't turn out that way. Brooke said, "It wasn't working for me when I dieted with the goal of getting thin. I could never stay on it and ended up feeling awful about myself. Why do I always fail at diets? Is there another way to eat, so I can feel better about myself?"*

To begin your journey to becoming an intuitive eater, the very first thing you need to know about is the first principle of Intuitive Eating—Reject the Diet Mentality. You'll learn why diets fail, how to get rid of the diet mentality, and why Intuitive Eating is so liberating and just the cure that every teen needs to heal from dieting.

activity 1 ✻ understanding the problem with diets

for you to know

I have a feeling you're thinking, "Well, what's wrong with diets? Why should I reject diet thinking?"

Let's look at why Brooke's dieting failed her. Here are some facts about the dangers of dieting (because you probably just love to be told all the reasons why something isn't good for you!):

- After restricting on a diet, you can become out of control when eating and feel that you don't know how to stop, making you feel helpless and powerless.

- Dieting can cause stress and feelings of failure, and lower your self-esteem and self-confidence.

- Dieting can lead to eating disorders.

- Dieting can increase social anxiety and wipe out your sense of self-trust.

- Diets reinforce body negativity, rather than promoting body positivity.

- Dieting can slow your metabolism.

- Almost all people who diet eventually can't stay on the diet and end up gaining back any weight they lost. And most of them go on to gain even more weight. So, dieting is a sure way to predict weight gain!

- Basically, dieting will make you miserable!

Doesn't that get you thinking that dieting is a pretty foolish thing to do? Or you might be thinking that those problems happen only in weak people and that you have great willpower. But even the most disciplined people who get their work done on time and don't get into trouble still can't stay on diets.

for you to do

If you've ever been on a formal diet—like Paleo or Weight Watchers, for example—or even one you've created, the following worksheet will help you remember why you started and stopped it, and your feelings while on it and afterward.

Write down your age when you went on your first diet, what type it was, and why you started it. Then, try to remember how you felt on the diet, how long you were able to stay on it, and why you dropped it. Finally, write about the feelings that came up when you quit it. Continue for any other diets you've been on. The first line shows Brooke's experience.

Age	Type of diet	Why did you start it?	Feelings on the diet	How long did you stay on it?	Why did you quit?	Feelings afterward
13	Low carb	Wanted to lose weight so I'd like myself more.	Excited, at first, then deprived, then frustrated.	Two weeks.	Couldn't keep it up. Started bingeing on carbs.	Felt like a failure, disappointed in myself. Unhappy.

more to do

In order to understand some of the feelings dieting has brought up for you, answer the following questions.

During or after a diet:	Yes	No
Have you had big cravings for carbohydrates?		
Have you felt out of control when satisfying these cravings?		
Have you felt the extreme hunger that happens when your blood sugar drops?		
Have you had mood swings?		
Have you had trouble sleeping?		
Have you felt overly tired?		
If you're a girl, have you missed a period (or more)?		
Have you noticed that you've lost hair or your hair is thinner?		
Do you avoid social situations where people are eating?		
If you eat with others, do you compare how much you eat to them?		
Are you self-conscious about eating with others?		
Have you ever counted calories (or fat grams or carbohydrate grams)?		
Do you feel guilty when you eat certain foods?		
Do you get distracted by thinking about how much you've eaten?		
Are you afraid you won't stop eating?		
Do you have "good" and "bad" food lists?		
Do you eat when stressed or bored?		
Do you eat when angry or lonely?		
Do you talk about dieting or food a lot?		
Do you avoid getting close to people?		

If you answered yes to any of these questions, you'll begin to understand the negative effects dieting has had on you. Write down any thoughts that came to you during this exercise.

_____

_____

_____

_____

_____

_____

_____

_____

activity 2 ✳ weighing the pros and cons of dieting

for you to know

Did you experience any negative feelings when you dieted (or maybe even some positive ones)? Do you think that dieting has done some harm to you? Making a pro and con list about how dieting has affected you can help you sort out your feelings and evaluate your experiences.

for you to do

In the pros column, write down any benefits you have ever felt that dieting has given you. For example, maybe it gave you the hope that you would lose weight and then have a perfect life.

Think about any negative effects dieting has had on your life, and list those in the cons column. For example, *"When I've been on a diet, I haven't wanted to go out for pizza with my friends, because I was afraid I'd lose my willpower and eat the forbidden pizza."* Or, *"Every time I've been on a diet, I can't stay on it for long and feel terrible about myself afterward."*

Pros of dieting	Cons of dieting

How many things did you put in the pros column and how many in the cons?

Pros _____ Cons _____

Which column had more? _____

more to do

As you look over your answers, write your thoughts about how dieting has affected you:

_____

_____

_____

_____

_____

_____

_____

activity 3 ✳ feeling the power of deprivation

for you to know

Have you ever been denied something you really wanted? (Of course you have; you're human, aren't you!) What happens when you want a car but can't afford one? Or when you have a crush on someone who doesn't like you back?

My hunch is that whatever you wanted and couldn't have has become really big and perfect and incredibly wonderful in your mind. You're probably thinking about it all the time and imagining how great your life would be if only you could have it. You're also probably having some very difficult feelings about not having it. Am I right?

The thoughts and feelings you're having have everything to do with the concept of deprivation. A psychologist named Abraham Maslow believed that we are driven by our unmet needs. In other words, we seek what we can't or don't have. What do you bet a homeless person is thinking about? Right—food for the next meal and shelter for the night. The power of deprivation is one of the main reasons why the instinctual part of you keeps diets from working.

for you to do

In this exercise, think about something you've wanted but couldn't get. Then, write about the feelings this brought up. The first line shows how Brooke answered this question.

What were you deprived of?	How did you feel?
Desperately wanted a dog, but my brother is allergic so I couldn't get one.	I felt sad and envious of my friends who had pets. I was also angry that I couldn't fix my brother's allergies.

more to do

A diet is the launching pad for deprivation. Whether the diet tells you not to eat cookies or candy or even bread, or it says to eat only chicken or fish and no red meat, the minute you hear one of these rules, all you can think about are the foods you're not supposed to eat.

Diets also tell you how much to eat. So, even if a diet doesn't take out any particular food (this is what Weight Watchers promotes), you're still going to feel deprivation, because you're allowed only a specific amount of certain foods. The minute you hear that you can have only two cookies or two pieces of bread or one small chicken breast or eighteen points (Weight Watchers, again), that creeping feeling of not getting to have enough pops right out of your head and into your mouth. Just thinking about not being able to have as much as you'd like opens the door to those feelings of deprivation.

Think about the possibility of not getting to have your favorite food or getting only a small amount of it. Here are some feelings that might come up. Mark the ones that fit for you, and use the blank lines to add others.

☐ Angry   ☐ Desirous

☐ Sad   ☐ Other: _____

☐ Frustrated   ☐ Other: _____

☐ Deprived   ☐ Other: _____

If you marked some of the feelings above, write the thoughts you now have about how food deprivation might affect you:

_____

_____

_____

_____

_____

activity 4 ✳ dieting leads to necessary rebellion

for you to know

I believe that diets are doomed to fail for another powerful, or even more powerful, reason than deprivation. It's the concept of rebellion.

Diets are like alien invaders. They find their way into the private place that holds all your information about hunger, fullness, what you like or don't like to eat, and how your body feels after you've eaten. It's normal and common for people to rebel against being told what to do, and that's exactly what happens with diets. You're given rules, which at some point will probably make you start to feel angry about having to follow them.

Oh, maybe at first, it sounds fun and exciting and even feels like your eating will get under control if you try the latest diet. In fact, going on a diet that all your friends are trying might even make you feel accepted and part of the crowd, but eventually you (and, by the way, everyone else) will start to feel rebellious and want to break these diet rules. You're bound to go off the diet and then feel bad about yourself for not being able to stay on it. But going off the diet is the inevitable result of feeling deprived and rebellious. It's not because you lack willpower!

The big question is, why do we feel rebellious when we're given rules and told what to do? Does it mean that we're just angry people or that we're like toddlers who have tantrums?

Well, in a certain way we do keep the feelings of a little kid in us throughout our lives. We do feel anger and want to tantrum when we're told no. When we were little, we didn't worry about what people thought. We just acted any way we wanted. If we felt angry, we cried or stomped our feet. We didn't have words to express difficult feelings. As we got older and began to speak and notice how people reacted when we screamed and yelled, we learned to put a cover on these feelings.

The truth is, these emotions are all normal, and all humans (and even cats and dogs) will feel them. This is because your healthy inner person is supposed to feel like making your own decisions. This is called *autonomy*. It means that you're an individual who isn't attached by an umbilical cord the way you were when your mother was pregnant with you. It means that as an individual, you want to make these decisions without anyone butting in.

In fact, your main job as a teenager is to find ways to be your own person. Sometimes this happens in ways that get you in trouble, like staying out past your curfew or hanging out with friends your parents don't like. You may do these things because it's hard to speak up and say, "I'm my own person, and I want to live my life the way I want." Or maybe you do express these things, and your parents tell you that they're the bosses, and as long as you're living in their house, you'll do what they say. But your parents are probably not trying to be mean. They likely set rules for you because they want to protect you from harm, and they're not sure that you'll make wise decisions for yourself. Their job is to notice when you do make wise decisions and, little by little, let you become an adult. In some homes, unfortunately, no one sits and listens to you or notices how grown-up you've become, which could make you feel very lonely. Sometimes, it's really hard being a teenager, isn't it?

for you to do

Do you remember any times when you rebelled against some rules your parents made? In this chart, write some of the rebellious acts you found yourself doing and then what the consequences were:

Rebellious act	Consequence

How did you feel after rebelling? Maybe you felt sorry about what you did because the consequences outweighed the benefits. Or maybe the powerful feeling you felt was worth the consequences. Write about these feelings below:

_____

_____

_____

_____

After exploring your feelings about any rebellious experiences you've had, you're ready to look at the role rebellion may have played if you have dieted.

more to do

Let's start by looking back at the history of dieting you completed in activity 1 to see some of the feelings you had when you couldn't stay on a diet.

Write the feeling below, and then mark whether it was due to deprivation, rebelliousness, or both:

Feeling	Due to deprivation	Due to rebelliousness	Due to both

What conclusions did you come to about the impact of deprivation and rebellion on your feelings when diets failed?

_____

_____

_____

_____

activity 5 ✳ intuitive eating is all about autonomy

for you to know

You might think it's strange that I'm telling you that being rebellious and needing to be autonomous is coming from a healthy part of you. But think of it this way—if you easily got sucked into a group that was doing things that didn't feel right to you and you couldn't find a way out, it would probably show that it's hard to have your own mind, which isn't so healthy.

A healthy, autonomous person is able to make decisions that aren't in reaction to other people or to please or hurt them. These decisions are rational and well thought out and don't make you feel bad about yourself afterward. That rebellious part of you is just longing to finally be able to make some decisions for yourself!

What is so cool about intuitive eating versus dieting is that with dieting, you're trying to obey other people's rules, and you're ultimately going to become rebellious. Eating intuitively, you get to make all your own decisions about eating, based on what your body is telling you. You are the only one in the world who knows what you like to eat, when you're hungry, when you're full, and how your body feels after eating a particular food. You don't have to wait to become an adult to listen to your inner wisdom about eating. At least this is one area where no one has a right to make decisions for you. In fact, it may be the only area in which you can be completely autonomous. You just need to be mindful so that you can hear your own words of wisdom.

for you to do

Write about how it might feel to be autonomous and be the expert on your eating.

_____

_____

_____

_____

activity 6 ✳ getting rid of the diet mentality

for you to know

Here are some actions that will help you start to become an intuitive eater:

- Get rid of your scale, or ask your parents to get rid of the scale in the house. Weighing yourself only gives power to the numbers on the scale, instead of to what your body knows about hunger and what satisfies your taste buds.

- Throw away any diet apps on your phone, like the ones that tell you the calories in foods or the fat or carb grams or how many calories you're burning when you exercise. Once again, they're an outside force that can begin to control you. This is all about trusting that your body knows how much you need. The numbers mean nothing compared to your body's inner smarts.

- Forget about measuring spoons or cups. As an intuitive eater, the only time you would ever need these is if you're cooking. Otherwise, they are simply diet tools!

- Most important, be kind to yourself. It isn't your fault that you've been sucked into diets and all their magical promises. You've been vulnerable to this as a way to deal with parts of your life that may be difficult to face. The most powerful word to use here is compassion. The more self-compassion you have, the lighter and happier you'll feel.

for you to do

List the tools you're willing to practice:

_____

_____

_____

_____

Which tool do you want to start with? _____

After you've conquered this tool, pick another when you're ready, until you've gone through the list. Are there others you think would help you?

_____

_____

_____

_____

Remember, listen to your inner wisdom, and come from the inside out, not the outside in! Since this may be the only part of your life where you're fully in charge, take it over in order to help you feel strong and independent. Isn't that what you're truly seeking?

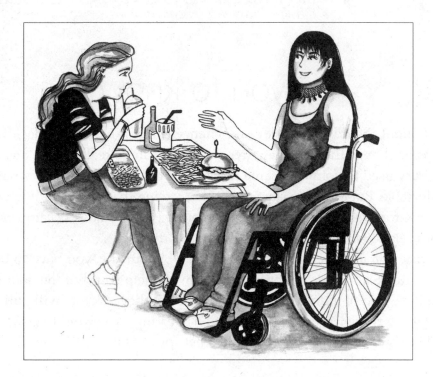

chapter 2

Savor and Be Satisfied!

After reading Chapter 1, I hope you're getting more pumped up about learning to be an intuitive eater. As you're trying to cross the threshold into intuitive eating, you may still have one little toe holding the door open to the world of dieting. This chapter is going to help you pull your whole foot into this new way of eating and slam that door forever, so dieting can never hurt you again.

Haley was very rigid in her eating. She said, "I was eating only clean foods—not the ones that hadn't fallen on the floor, but the ones I decided were the 'right' foods to eat—and never felt satisfied. I'm really getting sick of this depriving way of eating and wish that food could be more than fuel in your tank—I'd love to have some satisfaction when eating, too!"

When I used to diet, I never actually enjoyed my food. I never got to eat what I really wanted— it was always what I thought I should eat. Satisfaction in eating had completely flown out the door, and eating became simply about being "good" and staying on the diet. In this chapter, you'll learn another principle of Intuitive Eating: Discover the Satisfaction Factor. You'll explore the best way to find the most satisfying foods to eat and the best environment for your eating experience.

activity 7 ✳ what needs to change?

for you to know

Have you ever thought about why people make changes in their lives—say, deciding to get out of some friendships or change the way they dress? Change can be really scary, and a lot of people resist it. We get very used to doing the same thing the same way, because it's what we know and what feels comfortable. But often we start to get that feeling that whatever it is we're doing just isn't really working for us anymore. You may have picked up this book because you were feeling shaky about your relationship with food or were sick of dieting.

To take the risk of making any significant change in your life, you have to be motivated to find something better. So, what is it that's going to finally help you shut the door on dieting and land feet first in the world of intuitive eating? I believe that the hook that will pull you through is the promise of getting true pleasure and satisfaction in eating. Who wouldn't want that? Intuitive eating is actually founded on this promise, while diets prevent it!

for you to do

List the reasons you might want to change your relationship with food. Haley's first reason is: *"I need to find a way to enjoy food again!"*

_____

_____

_____

_____

_____

What feelings do you notice when you think about having more satisfying meals? Are you skeptical? Hopeful? Excited? Write about that here or in your journal.

_____

_____

_____

_____

_____

_____

_____

activity 8 ✳ choosing the foods you crave

for you to know

When people can't get or won't let themselves have the food they're really craving, they're left feeling disappointed. They may be physically full, but they begin to crave something else, looking for the satisfaction they didn't get from the wrong food. Rather than searching the cupboards afterward, getting the food you truly crave will lead you to a delicious, rewarding meal and a feeling of completeness.

for you to do

Think about a food you're particularly craving. Name it here:

_____

If you're able to get that food, after eating it, think about the pleasure it gave you. Describe what that felt like:

_____

_____

_____

_____

_____

If you weren't able to get the food you really wanted, did you eat something else instead? If so, how satisfying was it?

Very _____   Just okay _____   Not at all _____

How did you feel and what did you do after eating this substitute food? Perhaps you felt disappointed and went on to get something else to eat? Write about your experience here:

_____

_____

_____

_____

activity 9 ✱ why dieting is no fun

for you to know

If you've dieted, you've probably noticed that dieting takes away the pleasure of eating. This is mostly because you don't get to choose what you really want to eat. You're eating what the diet tells you to eat and you're forbidden from other foods. Only *you* know what foods truly please you—no diet can predict that! If you break the diet to eat what you're actually craving, whatever that is can't be very satisfying because you're so ridden with guilt for eating a forbidden food. Pleasure and guilt are two feelings that don't work well together!

for you to do

Think about the times you've dieted or held food restrictions. Do you remember whether you truly enjoyed your meals? On the lines that follow, write about whether you were satisfied when eating in this way, and why or why not.

_____

_____

_____

_____

_____

_____

_____

If you've come to the conclusion that dieting has taken the satisfaction out of eating for you, you can begin to feel the excitement of finding true eating pleasure.

Or not!

Do you have any thoughts or feelings about why you shouldn't be allowed to have meal satisfaction? If you have even a tiny feeling about this, it might be a good idea to talk to someone you trust about whether you feel worthy of receiving pleasure in life.

On the other hand, if you're completely with it on getting pleasure in your meals, there might be other barriers to letting satisfaction in. Perhaps you're thinking that if you really enjoy food, you might never want to stop eating? (Don't worry, we'll get to that in the next chapter.) Whatever fears or doubts you have will begin to disappear after doing the exercises in this and other chapters, and you'll be ready to take that leap into intuitive eating, because food is about to become one of the best pleasures in your life!

activity 10 ✳ finding a sense of satisfaction

for you to know

How do you decide what to eat when you're feeling hungry? Do you just go with the first thing that comes to your mind? Do you eat whatever is around? Do you choose your foods based on what you think you "should" be eating? Or do you eat what really sounds good?

To make eating more satisfying, you'll be exploring these various mouth and body sensations in this activity and the ones that follow:

taste	appearance
texture	body feel
temperature	staying power
aroma	

for you to do

In this exercise, you'll gather some feedback from your own body for a couple of these sensations. You'll get your best answers if you're mildly hungry.

The first sense to explore is *taste*. Put samples of foods on a plate to represent the five main tastes: sweet, salty, bitter, sour, and umami (savory or meaty); for example, a cookie, saltine cracker, radish, pickle, and piece of cooked hamburger.

Ask yourself, *What taste does my tongue really want?*

Here's a chart Haley used to explore taste:

What sense am I exploring?	I'm exploring what the taste buds on my tongue really want.
Which flavor did I pick?	Sweet
Which food did I sample?	A cookie
Was the taste pleasant?	Yes
Did it have the right amount of sweetness?	It was actually too sweet for me.
Did it satisfy me?	Almost—it would have been perfect if it were a little less sweet.

Now you try it. You can also download a copy to print at http://www.newharbinger.com/41443:

What sense am I exploring?	Taste
Which flavor did I pick?	
Which food did I sample?	
Was the taste pleasant?	
Did it have the right amount of _____? (Insert the flavor you picked.)	
Did it satisfy me?	

more to do

Here's a short exercise to help you start to explore *texture*. Go to http://www.newharbinger. com/41443 once again, and you'll find charts you can print and fill out to explore as many textures and other sensations as you like, including ones for temperature and aroma.

Draw a line from the following foods to their predominant texture (or textures):

Food	Texture
peanut butter	soft (gushy)
ice cream	crunchy
salad	lumpy
steak	smooth
tofu	silky smooth
bagel	chewy
mashed potatoes	sticky

activity 11 ✳ appearance can be appealing

for you to know

Have you seen any food commercials or cooking shows on television? Or maybe you've looked at food ads in magazines? The people who create these usually hire food stylists to set up the foods and food photographers to take photos of them, in order to make their *appearance* particularly appealing. Even someone posting a picture of food on Instagram will set it up to look inviting. They do this because they know that how the food looks can trigger someone's taste buds and desire to eat it.

for you to do

Cut out some pictures of food from magazines, or check out images of food on the internet, and print a few of them in color. (You might want to staple or glue them to a page in your notebook.) You can also take a picture on your phone of some of the meals you eat.

Which of the pictures look especially appealing to you?

_____

_____

What about them makes them look appealing?

_____

_____

Does your mouth start to water when you see a particular picture? Describe this picture:

_____

_____

Is there a picture that doesn't look appetizing? Why?

_____

_____

more to do

At http://www.newharbinger.com/41443, you'll find a blank chart you can use repeatedly to explore different food appearances, such as color, size, height, and arrangement. First, check out the one Haley filled out:

What sense am I exploring?	Appearance
Which appearance did I pick?	Varied colors
Which foods did I choose?	Spaghetti with red sauce and broccoli
Was the appearance pleasant?	Yes
Did it have the right amount of color variety?	Yes
Did it satisfy me?	Yes

Now it's your turn. Fill out the blank chart to decide whether the appearance of food is an important part of deciding what you want to eat.

What sense am I exploring?	
Which appearance did I pick?	
Which foods did I choose?	
Was the appearance pleasant?	
Did it have the right amount of _____ (insert the appearance you picked)?	
Did it satisfy me?	

activity 12 ✳ feeling body satisfaction

for you to know

The sensations of taste, texture, temperature, aroma, and appearance are all concentrated in your head. How your body feels, based on what you eat and what kind of staying power your food has, is also important to consider.

In thinking about how your body feels after different types of food or meals, one of the thoughts you might ponder is how long your body is satisfied after eating. There's that word "satisfied" again! You're beginning to see that satisfaction includes your tongue, your mind, and your body and how the different sensory aspects of food can bring you more or less satisfaction. Staying present and paying attention to all these aspects when you eat will allow you to savor your food in this quest.

for you to do

Download two more charts at http://www.newharbinger.com/41443 and fill them out to experiment with how certain foods make you feel and what their staying power is.

activity 13 ✱ planning a satisfying meal

for you to know

In searching for meal satisfaction, think about all your senses when you're trying to decide what to eat. Your body will offer a wealth of information if you practice tuning into its sensory messages about food.

for you to do

To help you pull it all together, ask the following questions to find a truly satisfying meal.

It's best if you do this when you are beginning to feel some hunger.

What taste does my tongue want to experience?	
What texture do I want to feel in my mouth?	
Which temperature would feel right?	
What aroma will be appealing to me?	
How do I want my food to look?	

How will my stomach feel after eating this meal?	
How long will my meal keep me satisfied before I get hungry again?	

What foods have you chosen?

_____

_____

Shortly after you begin eating, check in to see if the food meets your expectations. Describe the sensations you're experiencing.

_____

_____

Halfway through your meal, check in again to see if the meal still feels satisfying to all your senses. (Note: Scientists have found that the pleasantness of the sensory aspects of food actually begins to diminish after about two minutes of eating each food! Shocking, huh? This is called sensory-specific satiety.)

_____

_____

After you're finished, rate your satisfaction level on a scale of 1–5, with 1 being the least satisfying and 5 being the most. _____

Use these questions as often as you can when you're thinking about what to eat. At http://www.newharbinger.com/41443, you'll find a blank copy of the chart from this activity. It would be helpful to print as many copies as you like and save them in your notebook after you fill them out, so you can look back at them until this becomes automatic for you.

activity 14 ✳ exploring your eating environment: distractions and speed

for you to know

Now that you've become more conscious about picking just the right food(s) that will satisfy you, it's time to look at some other pieces of the satisfaction puzzle—the best ways to set up your eating environment to help maximize this satisfaction. The first is attention—and its enemy, distraction!

The second is how fast or slowly you eat. Inhaling your food will keep you from feeling the pleasure of your meal. Eating slowly will help you pay attention to all your senses and savor your meal. If you gobble it down, you won't get a chance to notice how good it tastes or whether the texture feels right in your mouth. One of the factors that can lead to fast eating is being in a big hurry and trying to "get through" eating. Sometimes, people don't want to take the time to focus on their meal, and instead, eat quickly, without real enjoyment. Eating in front of the fridge or standing over the sink means you're not letting yourself relax and pay attention to the sensory qualities of your food.

for you to do

The fewer distractions you have while eating, the more attention you'll give to your meals. Here are some distractions that can take away eating pleasure. Check the ones you sometimes do while eating:

☐ Talking on the phone

☐ Watching TV

☐ Being on social media

☐ Doing homework

☐ Reading a book or magazine

☐ Surfing the internet

☐ Driving a car

Are there any others?

_____

_____

_____

_____

_____

Which distractions are you willing to stop in order to find more meal satisfaction?

_____

_____

_____

_____

more to do

The next time you eat, keep your speed in mind. If you're a speed eater, try slowing down, and notice whether you get more satisfaction by being able to pay attention to all the sensory qualities of the food. If you're a slowpoke, you may find that the meal is less satisfying as it sits on your plate and gets cold.

What kind of eater are you most of the time?

Speed eater _____   Moderate eater _____   Slowpoke _____

How often do you eat in front of the fridge, over the sink, standing up, or on your way from one place to another?

Rarely _____   Sometimes _____   Often _____

Where do you tend to do this kind of eating, and when?

_____

_____

When people eat this way, they're usually rushed, and their focus is on anything but the experience of eating. If that's you, what could you do to change some habits that deprive you of satisfaction? For example, even if you can't get up earlier for breakfast, could you sit down while eating, instead of standing up?

_____

_____

_____

activity 15 ✳ exploring your eating environment: hunger and emotion

for you to know

Would you ever consider eating a peanut butter and jelly sandwich right before you go to your favorite restaurant for dinner? Probably not, because you know intuitively that eating that sandwich will spoil your enjoyment of your meal. And have you experienced going into a restaurant when you haven't eaten all day? If so, when the food arrives, you can't get it into your mouth fast enough!

Just as your level of hunger will affect how satisfying your meal is, what you're feeling emotionally can also have a big impact. Emotions and eating are deeply connected. Eating to push away or soothe feelings, rather than for hunger, might rob you of any chance to truly notice how wonderful your food can be.

for you to do

We'll talk more about hunger in a future chapter, but for now, start noticing: do you get more satisfaction from a meal if you're ravenous? Moderately hungry? Not hungry at all?

Pick a meal to practice the following exercise:

What foods are in your meal? _____

_____

_____

How hungry are you?

Ravenous _____   Moderately hungry _____   Not hungry _____

When you've finished eating, ask yourself: was the meal satisfying?

Yes _____   No _____

Reflect on whether your meal was as satisfying as you had hoped, and why (or why not):

_____

_____

_____

_____

_____

_____

If you noticed that you got more satisfaction by starting your meal when you were moderately hungry, remember to wait to eat until you feel this hunger level, but not too long that you feel so empty that you worry there can't be enough food to fill this bottomless pit!

more to do

We're going to have a whole chapter to explore emotional eating, but since it's part of your environment, we'll check in about it here, too.

Do you think that you may sometimes be an emotional eater? If so, check the emotions that might make you want to eat when you're not hungry:

☐ Boredom

☐ Loneliness

☐ Anxiety

☐ Anger

☐ Fear

☐ Sadness

☐ Any others?

_____

_____

_____

If you've found that you do eat emotionally at times, stay tuned for tools to change this later in this workbook.

activity 16 ✳ exploring your eating environment: conflict and chaos

for you to know

For many people, nothing kills enjoyment in a meal more than trying to eat when there's conflict going on—whether you're arguing with someone, or others near you are arguing.

For others, the state of their surroundings while eating can also make a difference in how satisfying their meal is. Tidy, pretty, peaceful surroundings increase satisfaction, while chaos and mess make mealtimes miserable.

for you to do

If you've ever experienced trying to eat in a room full of anger and argument, describe it here. Consider what feelings you had. How do you think they affected your meal satisfaction?

_____

_____

_____

_____

Can you think of some ways to avoid these situations in the future or to find some inner calm while in the midst of them? For example, could you put your food in the fridge until there's peace again in your world?

_____

_____

_____

If there's no way to avoid the conflict that surrounds you, try closing your eyes and taking a few deep breaths before eating. It will help quiet your mind and body and distance you from the conflict. At school, could you find a more peaceful place to eat than the loud cafeteria?

_____

_____

_____

more to do

Imagine sitting down to eat your dinner at a table that has a nice placemat, pretty dishes, and some space to spread out. How does that sound to you?

_____

Now, imagine throwing a bunch of papers all over the table and putting a paper towel under your dish instead of a placemat. Instead of nice silverware, picture a plastic fork with a broken prong next to your plate, and, oh, to make it even more chaotic, imagine some construction noise next door. How satisfying do you think your meal would be under these conditions?

_____

_____

Eating in a pleasant space with some favorite music playing or simply in a quiet room can give you a much better chance of having a satisfying eating experience. Here are some ideas to help you achieve these goals:

- If it feels comfortable for you, let your family know that you'd like their help in making meals more enjoyable.

- Offer to help by setting the table in a way that looks good to you.

- Ask if it would be okay to put some music on while eating.

- At school, try to find a quiet corner of the cafeteria to eat lunch with a good friend.

- If you're eating alone, put your headset on and listen to music that calms you.

How could you change your eating environment to have more pleasurable meals?

Home: _____

_____

_____

_____

School: _____

_____

_____

_____

In other places: _____

_____

_____

_____

activity 17 ✳ satisfaction: seeing the big picture

for you to know

It's your right to have satisfaction in your eating and to explore ways to find it. The way I see it, satisfaction is the driving force of intuitive eating. If you've got your eye on satisfaction, you'll want to pick the foods you most enjoy and savor them by staying present to all their sensory qualities. You'll pay attention to eating when you're moderately hungry and, if you can, when you're emotionally calm. And if your environment is set up in an appealing way, you've hit the bull's-eye of pleasurable eating.

for you to do

Now it's time for you to take all the pieces of the puzzle and put them together, so that you can create meals and an environment that give you the most pleasure and satisfaction in your eating world.

Use the following worksheet to rate the factors that can either give you the most satisfaction while eating or take it away. The next time you sit down to eat a meal, evaluate any of the environmental factors listed below that apply. Then circle the word that mostly describes your experience. Finally, rate your satisfaction on a scale of 1–5, with 1 being a very unsatisfying meal, and 5 meaning that your meal has put a happy smile on your face! Use the final column to add any comments.

Satisfaction factors	Your experience	Satisfaction rating (Scale of 1–5)	Comments
Speed of eating	Fast Medium Slow		
Staying present	Yes or No		
Eating when distracted	Yes or No		
Eating when ravenous	Yes or No		
Eating when not hungry	Yes or No		
Eating when moderately hungry	Yes or No		
Eating with tension in the room	Yes or No		
Eating in peace	Yes or No		
Eating in a chaotic space	Yes or No		
Eating in a pleasant space	Yes or No		
Standing while eating	Yes or No		

Sitting while eating	Yes or No		
Eating with negative emotions	Yes or No		
Eating when feeling good	Yes or No		

Which factors gave you the highest satisfaction ratings?

_____

_____

Which had the lowest ratings?

_____

_____

Which of the low-scoring factors would you like to focus on changing, and what are the first steps you can take toward reaching this goal?

_____

_____

_____

_____

You can download this chart at http://www.newharbinger.com/41443 to use over and over to explore all the environmental factors that affect a meal.

more to do

Now that you've reviewed your eating environment, take a moment to think about all the sensations you've explored that make eating such an enjoyable part of your life. Number these sensations from 1 to 7 in the order that's most important to you. For example, some people think taste is the number one sensation that makes or breaks their meals. For others, it's whether their meal will give them enough energy to get through a sport or activity and not leave them feeling starved afterward.

Sensation	Order of importance (1–7)
Taste	
Texture	
Temperature	
Aroma	
Appearance	
Body feel	
Staying power	

Describe the most interesting or newest insight you discovered by doing the activities in this chapter.

_____

_____

_____

_____

_____

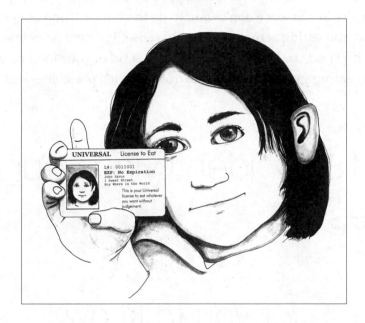

chapter 3

Your License to Eat
What You Like

Getting your first driver's license has to rank as one of the most liberating experiences of your life. A world of freedom suddenly opens up to you when you don't have to depend on someone always driving you around. In a similar way, giving yourself license to eat whatever you like, without "good" and "bad" foods or food rules, will free up your relationship with food and release you from Food Jail.

> *Laura, a high school student who was looking for this freedom, said, "When I went to camp last summer, I never let myself eat the fun foods all my friends were eating. I always felt deprived, but I never gave in because I wanted to be healthy. When I came home, I couldn't stop eating the foods I didn't allow myself that summer. I want to work on throwing out all my forbidden-food ideas and see if that helps me stop overeating. I want to feel free!"*

Laura was living by a set of rules she created for herself. She, like you, has been bombarded by messages about when and how much to eat, about good foods and bad foods, about foods that will help you live forever and those that could kill you tomorrow, about foods that will help you get the body you want and those that will make you hate your body and yourself. These messages can lead to food rules that can make you feel trapped and feel as if you're living in Food Jail.

We often follow rules because we don't want to do the wrong thing or get into trouble, but creating rules about food and eating actually makes no sense. The next principle of Intuitive Eating is called Make Peace with Food, and you'll learn how to get rid of your food rules and have the same emotional reaction to eating gummy bears or carrots. Yes, it's possible—and I'll show you how!

activity 18 ✳ identifying your food rules

for you to know

The only way you'll be able to make peace with food is to identify the food rules you've been carrying around so that you can ultimately throw them all out.

Some of the rules people try to live by include:

- Don't eat carbs because they're fattening.

- Don't eat anything after six p.m.

- Don't mix protein with carbs.

I'm sure you've noticed the one word that's in all these examples. Right—it's "don't"! As you learned in the first chapter, any time we're given rules, it's our natural tendency to feel rebellious about being told what to do.

for you to do

First, let's get a handle on your food rules. For each rule in the table that follows, put an X under "Yes" or "No." Use the empty boxes to add any of your own personal rules. (Laura put an X by numbers 3, 6, and 13.)

Yes	No	Food rules
		1. I have rules about the times that I eat.
		2. I don't allow myself to eat certain foods.
		3. I eat certain foods only when I'm with friends who are eating them.
		4. I have rules around what beverages I drink.
		5. I let myself have sweets only on special occasions.
		6. I don't let myself eat fried foods.
		7. I often compare what I eat to what others eat.
		8. I throw out my food rules on weekends.
		9. I don't let myself snack between meals.
		10. I try to wait as long as I can before eating anything after I get up.
		11. I eat very little during the day so I can eat more at night.
		12. I let myself eat a forbidden food only if I exercise that day.
		13. I eat only foods that I think are healthy.
		14. I have rules about the amounts of foods I let myself eat.
		15. I count calories and allow myself only a certain number each day.
		16. I count fat or carb grams and have a rule about how many I should eat each day.
		17.
		18.
		19.
		20.

If you follow any food rule, describe how you follow it, how it affects you, and how you feel about it. For example, Steve, another high school student, follows Rule 9—I don't let myself snack between meals. Here's what he wrote: *"I come home from school and start my homework, but sometimes I get so hungry that I can't concentrate and start daydreaming until dinner. I feel good that I'm keeping my rule, but, boy, do I feel lousy, and once I start eating dinner, there's never enough food to fill me up."*

Food rule: _____

How do you follow it?

_____

_____

_____

How does this affect you?

_____

_____

_____

How do you feel about holding on to this food rule?

_____

_____

_____

_____

Continue in your notebook with the rest of your food rules.

activity 19 ✱ recognizing where your food rules come from

for you to know

Any food rules that drive your eating had to come from somewhere, because you weren't born with them! Think about where they may have started. Did your family have a lot of rules? Are you listening to your friends' rules? Do you read posts on social media that tell you what to eat, how much to eat, or even when to eat?

Perhaps in your family you were told to finish everything on your plate, or you were told that you couldn't have dessert until you finished your meal or only on the weekends. Maybe your friends talk about foods they avoid in order to lose weight. Or are you following people who post about "clean eating," or reading about celebrities' food rules?

for you to do

This worksheet will help you find the source of your food rules. Write a food rule you hold in the first column. Then put an X in the column that describes what or who influenced this rule. Continue with other rules and mark their source. The first row shows Laura's responses.

Food rule	Influence				
	Family	Friends	Social media or magazines	Television or movies	Other source
I let myself have sweets only on special occasions.	X	X	X		

more to do

Take one of the food rules you identified above. Use the space below to write about the influences that have prompted your food rule and how you feel about it.

_____

_____

_____

_____

_____

_____

_____

_____

In your notebook, do this exploration of your other food rules.

activity 20 ✳ breaking your food rules—and letting them go

for you to know

You now know that you weren't born with your food rules, that they were influenced by outside sources, and that the healthy part of you is bound to reject them. It doesn't matter whether you hold them as part of a diet or for health reasons; food rules will ultimately fail because they're not aligned with your inner world. No baby has a rule that says, "I'll drink only eight ounces of milk and will wait four hours before I cry for more." No way! That baby goes by innate signals of hunger and fullness in order to begin and stop eating.

There is nothing about food rules that will make you happy. They'll only make you feel resentful or deprived and ultimately bad about yourself. Letting go of them is your first step toward eating freedom.

for you to do

In the space below, write down some of your food rules you've broken and how you felt afterward. Laura's example is in the first row. If you need more space, take this activity to your notebook.

Broken food rule	How you felt after breaking it
I let myself have sweets only on special occasions.	When I couldn't resist sweets at friends' houses or at school, I felt like a failure.

more to do

Even if they sound good or wise or healthy, all food rules keep you from tuning into your intuitive wisdom about eating. If you maintain your old food rules or make new ones, they're bound to fail. So, the first step in making peace with food is to throw your rules out the window.

Using the list of food rules you identified in activity 18, write down any you might be willing to let go:

_____

_____

_____

_____

_____

What thoughts and feelings come up when you think about releasing each of these rules? (Take it to your notebook if you need more space.)

_____

_____

_____

_____

_____

You've learned why keeping food rules just doesn't make sense, but sometimes it's really hard to let them go. Do you have any fears that might keep you from breaking free? Here are some common fears that teens (and adults, too) carry around:

"If I stop following rules and just let myself eat whatever I want, I'll never stop eating it."

"If I eat whatever I want, I'll only choose junk food."

"If I eat what I want and my friends are following rules, I won't fit in."

List any fears you have that you think may be reinforcing your food rules:

_____

_____

_____

_____

_____

In the next activities, you'll learn some reasons why food fears are unfounded.

activity 21 ✳ understanding habituation

for you to know

Have you ever imagined spending time with someone who seems beyond your reach, and then your dream comes true? At first you feel thrilled, but my hunch is that after a few months, or maybe even a few weeks, the excitement burns out. And maybe after you get to know them, you don't even like them at all! If this sounds familiar, you've experienced *habituation*—the tendency our brains have to want less of a thing, the more of it we have.

The same goes for food. The mere thought of any food you've forbidden can make you feel super excited. But once you have full permission to eat it whenever you want, forever, it loses the thrill, and you can actually get sick of it. That happened with a client of mine who tried this out with grilled cheese sandwiches. She committed to having one a day for a week. The following week, I asked how it went. Instead of being in bliss, she said that after the third day, she couldn't even look at another grilled cheese!

for you to do

In the chart that follows, list some of your forbidden foods in the first column. Then give yourself permission to eat as much of one of them as you want each day for a week. (In the next chapter, we'll talk about what to do if your parents give you flak about your eating. If they do, for the time being, just tell them that it's an exercise you've been asked to do in your workbook.) In the second column, rate how amazing the food tasted on the first bite, with 5 being super incredible. In the last column, note how long it took for the excitement to wear off and the food to taste ordinary.

But before you begin, there's one very important caution to keep in mind. If you haven't actually given yourself full permission to eat this food forever and plan to forbid it again in the future, the experience will backfire. Even the tiniest thought of future deprivation will prevent habituation from happening. You have to be fully committed to permanently legalizing this food for the excitement to fade away and the food to become just an ordinary part of your life.

Previously forbidden food	How amazing was the first bite? (Scale of 1–5)	How many days before the excitement began to wear off?

Pick one of the forbidden foods you allowed yourself to eat. When you first bit into it, how excited were you to eat it and how amazing did it taste?

_____

_____

_____

_____

Describe your experience throughout the week. When did habituation start to set in? For example, did you notice that the thrill started to wear off after three days? Or did it take longer (or shorter) for this to happen?

_____

_____

_____

_____

Continue this exercise with each of the foods you listed. Understanding habituation will help you trust that it's unfounded that you'll _never_ stop eating any particular food. In fact, you may soon get sick of it!

Note: When you first begin to give yourself license to eat what you like, you may find that you eat more of the foods you used to forbid, and you might eat them more often. For a while, that is! Just the whole idea of having this kind of freedom can be very exhilarating, but just like the excitement of each food will wear off, so will the excitement of having this freedom. It will become just a regular part of your eating life.

activity 22 ✻ tracking what you eat for a week

for you to know

"If I eat whatever I want, I'll choose only junk food" is a common food fear. First of all, we're going to throw the term "junk food" right in the garbage can where it belongs—the term that is, not the food! To me, there's no such thing as junk food. I like to call it "play food," and I'll talk more about my reasons for that in a later chapter.

Scientists who have studied toddlers' eating habits have found that if they are given a wide variety of foods—very nutritious foods, along with play foods—within a week, they'll eat many different types of foods and get all the nutrition they need. They might eat a lot of macaroni and cheese one day and want tons of strawberries and carrots the next.

for you to do

Be your own scientist. For a week, collect data on what you eat. You'll find a sample food record below followed by a blank chart. You can copy the blank chart or at http://www.newharbinger.com/41443, you'll find a chart you can download. For one week, write down everything you eat and drink each day. Note the time you eat, and use general amounts (for example, a medium burger rather than a six-ounce burger) and as many food categories per meal as needed. (You'll learn more about these food categories in the nutrition chapter.)

Here are some examples of foods within various categories:

- Proteins—meat, poultry, fish, shellfish, beans, nuts, eggs, dairy

- Carbohydrates—bread, cereal, pasta, popcorn, potatoes, cookies, rice, sweet potatoes

- Fats—butter, oil, salad dressing, avocado, mayonnaise, cream

- Fruits and vegetables—apple, orange, banana, grapes, fruit juice, salad, carrots, broccoli

- Dairy—milk, yogurt, cheese, ice cream, frozen yogurt

- Play foods—chips, fries, cookies, candy, cake, donuts, soda

- Beverages—water, coffee, milk, tea

Time	Food and drink	Amount (approximate)	Category
7:00 a.m.	Cheerios and milk Orange juice	Medium bowl One small glass	Carbs, protein, dairy, fruit
10:00 a.m.	Power bar	One	Protein, carbs, fat
12:00 p.m.	Turkey sandwich on whole wheat bread with mayo Chips Apple Water	Two slices of bread A few slices of turkey Small bag of chips Medium apple One bottle	Carbs, protein, fat, fruit, play food, beverage
3:00 p.m.	String cheese Grapes Chocolate chip cookies Milk	One cheese Bunch of grapes Two medium cookies One medium glass	Protein, carbs, fat, dairy, fruit, play food
5:00 p.m.	Fruit smoothie	Large glass	Protein, fruit
7:30 p.m.	Salad Cheeseburger with bun Broccoli	Medium bowl Medium burger, one bun Two stalks broccoli	Protein, carbs, fat, dairy, vegetables
10:00 p.m.	Ice cream	Two medium scoops	Protein, fat, dairy

Time	Food and drink	Amount (approximate)	Category

At the end of the week, list the foods you ate within each category in the first column of the chart that follows. Put a mark in the second column every time you ate a food in each category. In the last column, total the servings of food per category. When Laura filled out the chart, she found that she ate chicken three times, red meat twice, turkey four times, fish once, beans once, eggs three times, and cheese five times. When she added up her protein foods, she found that she had eaten nineteen servings of protein in a week.

Foods you ate in each category	How many times?	How many total servings in the week?
Proteins		
Carbohydrates		
Fats		
Fruits and vegetables		
Dairy		
Play foods		
Beverages		
Total		

Did you eat something from each of the food groups mentioned above? _____

If not, which was missing? _____

Did you find that you ate multiple servings from many of the food groups? _____

Which groups were these?

_____

_____

_____

_____

_____

Were there any groups where you'd like to add more foods? _____

Which are these?

_____

_____

_____

_____

Can you conclude that you ate a variety of foods during the week? _____

If so, it's likely that you've made peace with all foods.

activity 23 ✱ food rules and friends

for you to know

It's always hard to be the maverick—the one who does what feels personally right and doesn't always get led by the crowd. You may share this common fear mentioned earlier: "If I eat what I want and my friends are following rules, I won't fit in."

for you to do

Name some of the ways you can fit in with your friends that don't include food; for example, wearing some of the same styles of clothes or listening to the same bands.

_____

_____

_____

_____

_____

Being an intuitive eater is unique in a world of food rules, dieting, and judgment about size or shape. It's also a way to feel independent, knowing that you have a mind of your own. Randy hangs out with friends from his baseball team on weekends and some weeknights. Some of his friends live on pizza, fries, and sodas when they're not home, but he's found that others talk "diet talk" they've learned from their trainer. The diet-talk guys think they should eat only oatmeal, egg whites, chicken breasts, fruits, and veggies. Sometimes, Randy feels that he doesn't fit into either group. He loves pizza and play food, but when he goes out with the pizza guys too often, he misses some of the more nutritious foods he likes. When he's out with the diet-talk guys, he feels self-conscious if he orders a burger and fries.

In the lines below, write about your experience of wanting to go along with your friends, but knowing that it doesn't fit into your ideas about eating. Identify any people, places, or situations that were particularly challenging. If there were any food rules that others followed, how did that affect you?

_____

_____

_____

_____

_____

_____

_____

_____

_____

_____

The truth is that real friends will like you, even if you don't do exactly what they do. If you're true to your taste buds and stop judging foods, the pleasure you'll find in eating will outweigh the feelings of not fitting in. You're likely to find that your friends don't really care what you eat, and you might even end up having a positive influence on freeing them from their food rules. And the biggest benefit is less stress around eating and way more pleasure!

activity 24 ✳ exploring your favorite foods

for you to know

I once asked a client what her favorite foods were. There was stunned silence for a long time. She finally said, "I haven't a clue about what foods I like. I only know which I shouldn't eat, because I was always told they were bad. And if I ever broke down and ate any of them, I couldn't stop eating, because I felt so guilty and just knew I would never let myself eat them again."

Her assignment was to spend a week paying attention to the foods she actually liked and to eat them with full permission. When she returned, she said that she had found only nine foods she really liked, and her favorite was Wonder Bread (a bread that starts out really soft, can be rolled up in a ball, getting sticky and kind of hard). This didn't sound very exciting to me, but everyone has a right to a favorite. She actually spent a couple of days eating only Wonder Bread! When I asked her how that was for her, she said, "I felt really crappy and realized that I needed some protein!" That discovery was her first moment of intuitive eating, and she loved the freedom she felt.

for you to do

Explore your favorite foods, without judgment or guilt. In the first column, list all your favorite foods. In the next column, put a check by the ones you'd like to eat the next time you're hungry. After you've eaten the food, write about how this experience turned out. For example,

Did you actually enjoy the food?

Did it satisfy your taste buds and your body?

Did you have any lingering feelings of judgment or guilt?

Will you eat this food whenever you crave it?

Were you disappointed?

In the first row, you'll see what Laura's experience was when she tried this exercise.

Favorite foods	✓	How was your experience?
Potato chips	✓	They were yummy at first, but after I kept eating them, I kind of got sick of them. Maybe they'd taste good with a sandwich next time I want them, rather than eating them by themselves.

At the end of this exercise, you might find that some of the foods you thought you loved (and maybe didn't allow yourself to eat very often) turned out to be disappointing. Others might truly be your favorites. The more you stay present while tasting your food, the better your opportunity to keep the foods you love and ditch the ones you don't.

And one last thing—stay aware of whether you're eating certain foods just to prove to yourself that you can. I promise—your license will never be revoked!

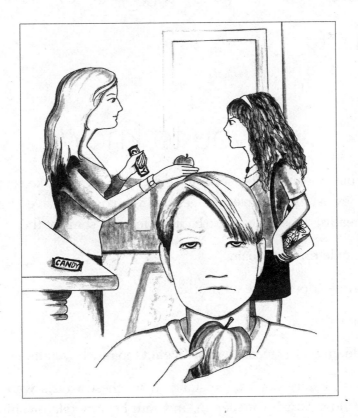

chapter 4

Banishing the Food Police

You may still have some negative food thoughts despite all the work you've done on food rules and where they came from. These thoughts are being spoken by an old voice that has taken residence in your mind. You can think of this voice as coming from something called the "Food Police," who just love to catch you and make you feel bad about your eating or your body.

Ben told me, "My parents notice every bite of food I put in my mouth. There are only 'healthy' foods in my house, and when we go to a restaurant, they don't let me order fries or dessert. I feel like I'm in Food Jail, and they're the Food Police. I'm so frustrated!"

Another principle of Intuitive Eating is called Challenge the Food Police. In this chapter, you'll learn about the ways the Food Police make you feel bad and try to keep you in Food Jail, and how to rid your life of them forever!

activity 25 ✳ spotting the food police

for you to know

For some unexplainable reason, people seem to think it's okay to make comments about others' size, shape, or what they eat. If you have younger siblings, you may have heard people remarking about their bodies or eating when they were babies. Here are some of them:

- "What an adorable roly-poly baby!"

- "Oh, she's so tiny—doesn't she eat much?"

- "Wow, that baby can eat a lot!"

- "Better slow down on the feeding, or he'll gain too much weight."

Fortunately, because babies don't understand them, these words won't have an impact on them. But once you're older, words can seep in, and your healthy relationship with food and your body is likely to start unraveling.

The people making these statements are speaking the words of the external Food Police. Here are some comments you may have heard about yourself:

- "You've gotten so much bigger since I saw you last."

- "Have you thought about working out at a gym? You could build some muscle and tighten up your body that way."

- "Haven't you had enough to eat?"

- "What's wrong with you for eating so much sugar?"

- "Better watch those carbs—carbs can put on weight."

- "Don't eat anything after six p.m., because all you do is sit around and then go to sleep."

No one has a right to make these kinds of judgmental statements! If the external Food Police show up and start talking about your body or telling you what you can and can't eat or how much you "should" eat, their words will be soaked up by you and stored somewhere inside, becoming the voice of the internal Food Police. Notice how easily the external Food Police can transform into your own critical voice. When you're feeling bad about something—boom!—the internal Food Police appear to make you feel even worse.

for you to do

If you can remember something negative that was said to you about eating or your body when you were younger, write down your approximate age in the first column below. Then write the comment, who made it and, if you remember, how you felt afterward and/or how the memory of it makes you feel now.

One of the negative comments made to Ben is below.

Age	Comment	Who made the comment	Feelings then and/or now
13	Better watch those carbs—carbs can put on weight.	My mother	I felt so bad then, and her judgment still stays with me now and makes me feel bad when I eat carbs!

Remembering what the Food Police said to you when you were younger, describe how this may affect your life now.

_____

_____

_____

_____

_____

activity 26 ✳ challenging the food police: getting started

for you to know

Our thoughts can have a powerful effect on our feelings. Negative or judgmental thoughts can make us feel terrible about ourselves. Challenging those thoughts and realizing they're not helpful can lift our spirits. Keep in mind that you didn't invent them. They're not part of your inner wisdom, so what's the point of holding on to them?

Just because you have a thought doesn't mean it's a fact. You'll be able to know that a thought comes from the Food Police by how you feel when you hear it. Do you feel uncomfortable, uneasy, upset, angry, or rebellious? These may be the same feelings you had when the external Food Police spoke to you as a child or speak to you now as a teenager. If you're feeling imprisoned by the Food Police, it's time to begin challenging what they're telling you. If you don't, you won't feel the peace that comes with intuitive eating.

The first step is to understand that these thoughts came from the external Food Police and stem from toxic myths that create the negative belief systems floating around in our society. Some beliefs include the culturally thin or buff ideal, "good" and "bad" foods, and the "value" of dieting. Eventually, the external Food Police statements and commands turn into the internal Food Police and can gang up together to lock you right up in Food Jail.

for you to do

If the Food Police live in your head, write down some of the things they say to you and how they make you feel. Here are some examples of their words:

- "You eat way too much. You have no control!"

- "You're always wanting sweets—what's wrong with you?"

- "Why can't you ever just want raw vegetables?"

Internal Food Police statement	How it makes you feel

The sad thing about the Food Police is that after listening to a lot of what they have to say about you, you soon start to believe them and begin to lose trust in your inner wisdom.

Here are some steps for challenging the internal Food Police:

1. From your list above, choose a Food Police thought:

    _____

    _____

2. Ask yourself how holding on to this thought is helping you.

    If you decide it's not helping you, you can challenge it by having some responses ready for the Food Police. For example:

    a. "Oh no, you're not going to control me."

    b. "I'll trust the inner wisdom I was born with to tell me how to eat—not you!"

    c. "I think that all foods are allowed and legal, so buzz off."

    Write some responses you might come up with:

    _____

    _____

    _____

    _____

    _____

3. Try doing the opposite of what the Food Police tells you. For example:

    *   If the Food Police tell you not to eat carbs, make yourself a sandwich or a bowl of pasta.

    *   If they tell you that you can eat dessert only once a week and not until after dinner, try eating dessert for your meal.

    What opposite actions could you take?

    _____

    _____

    _____

How did it feel to defy the command of the Food Police? Maybe you felt great for doing what you really wanted to do. If instead, you felt guilty, you might want to reread the previous chapter on making peace with all foods.

_____

_____

_____

_____

_____

_____

activity 27 ✳ challenging the food police: banishing black-and-white thinking

for you to know

The Food Police love to tell you to _never_ do something or _always_ do something. When you hear either of these words, you're hearing a _black-and-white statement_. This kind of thinking is based on rules that are likely to be broken and to lead you to feeling bad. When you learn to notice these statements around food, you'll be able to identify them as the rule-based words of the Food Police.

for you to do

You can change your own black-and-white statements to something more reasonable. For example, "I should never eat sweets" can be changed to "I can eat sweets when I know I'll enjoy them."

Notice or remember some black-and-white statements about food that you may be in the habit of making. Write them below. Counter each one with a restatement that is reasonable and true and doesn't set you up for failure. The first row shows you how Ben did this.

Black-and-white statement	Reasonable restatement
I should eat vegetables every day.	I'll try to add some vegetables I like when they're available. I'll probably eat plenty during the week.

activity 28 ✳ challenging the food police: the trap of perfectionism

for you to know

Are you someone who is usually trying to get the best grade, run the fastest mile, or hang out with only the most popular kids? Perfectionism is a real trap related to black-and-white thinking. It keeps you striving for something that is actually impossible to achieve, and that failure can keep you from trying things you're not sure you can do perfectly. Physicist Albert Einstein said, "A person who never made a mistake never tried anything new."

for you to do

In what ways are you trying to be perfect in the realm of food and eating? (Hint: This can even happen with the tools and insights you're learning in this workbook.) For example, Ben was excited about how having satisfying meals would give him a better relationship with food. He promised himself, "I'll only eat satisfying meals from now on!" Watch out for words like "always," "never," and "only."

Write one or two ways you try to be perfect around food and eating:

_____

_____

_____

_____

activity 29 ✳ challenging the food police: using "for the most part" thinking

for you to know

One way out of perfectionist thinking is to use the phrase "for the most part." When you say this, you give yourself the chance to set an intention to do the best you can do in some area. For example, Ben might say, "For the most part, I'm going to find a way to have satisfying meals." This leaves room for times when he might have to eat on the run or eat something that isn't his first choice because it's all that's around.

In challenging the Food Police, you could say, "I'm going to set the goal, for the most part, to make positive statements about food or my body. If a negative statement happens to sneak in, I can notice it in a neutral way, without getting disappointed in myself. After all, none of us is perfect!"

for you to do

Pick one area where you've been trying to be perfect, and let the goal of perfection go. To work on doing your best without thinking it has to be perfect, incorporate the term "for the most part" in your answer.

_____

_____

_____

The more you work on letting go of the goal of perfectionism, the better chance you have of releasing your Food Police thoughts.

activity 30 ✱ exploring how your feelings affect your actions

for you to know

Just as thoughts can have a powerful effect on your feelings, feelings can equally impact your actions. Often, when people start to feel bad about their food or bodies, they can end up:

Avoiding social situations or activities they love. For example—not going out to eat with your friends because you're afraid you might break a Food Police rule, or deciding not to go to the beach because the Food Police are telling you your body isn't good enough to be in a bathing suit.

Deciding to go on a diet or restrict certain foods, in order to try to change their body. Negative Food Police comments can make you feel frustrated with yourself and make you beat yourself up emotionally. Hearing promises that diets can help you lose weight and change your life can be very enticing. But you know how that story ends!

By challenging the Food Police with positive thoughts, you'll feel better and get the chance to have fun, enjoy life, and have satisfying eating experiences.

for you to do

Here are some examples of actions you can take that show you're feeling better and challenging the Food Police.

- If the Food Police tell you not to go swimming until you eat less and lose weight, make a plan to go to a pool or beach with friends who make neutral or positive comments about themselves and others.

- If you hear people making statements that come from the Food Police, change the subject to anything other than food. Talk about music you like, a movie you saw, or a vacation you'd like to take.

- Unfollow people on Instagram who post memes about good or bad foods or pictures of themselves showing off their bodies.

What other actions can you take to show that you're challenging the Food Police?

1. _____

_____

_____

2. _____

_____

_____

3. _____

_____

_____

activity 31 ✳ speaking up for yourself

for you to know

You've worked hard at identifying your internal Food Police and finding ways to change your belief system and thoughts in order to release yourself from Food Jail. But there's one more job you need to do in order to feel fully free. That job is to practice speaking up to the external Food Police. This job can be scarier than speaking up to your own voice. You might be afraid that people will get angry at you for saying what you think and might even punish you.

There's a term for not speaking up: self-silencing. Intuitive eaters do less self-silencing than people who go on diets. They are more likely to take the risk of speaking up, because they love how it feels to be independent and stand up for what they believe.

for you to do

Melanie's mother regularly brags about how she keeps her weight down by exercising excessively and "eating right." She tells Melanie that if she would only do the same, she could have a body like hers. Melanie is afraid to speak up and self-silences her deep feelings of not being accepted because she knows her mother will never understand.

Name two or three areas of your eating and body-image life where you self-silence.

_____

_____

_____

_____

_____

What fears do you have about speaking your own truth?

_____

_____

_____

_____

_____

Here are some statements you can practice when you feel strong enough to speak up for what you believe:

- "I believe that my body is very wise and that I can depend on it to tell me how to eat."

- "If I listen to all the messages about good and bad foods, I end up feeling bad about myself if I don't choose the 'good' foods. I don't want to feel that way anymore."

- "This is my body, and I have a right to decide what foods I put into it."

- "I'm not going to buy into the belief that everyone should look one way, and I'm not going to diet to try to change my body."

What are some other statements you could make when you're ready?

_____

_____

82

_____

_____

more to do

Practice speaking up to a person in your life who seems safe.

Who is it? _____

What do you want to say?

_____

_____

_____

_____

_____

After you've spoken up, write about how it went for you to say what you really believe. How did the person react, and how did you feel afterward?

_____

_____

_____

_____

_____

Congratulations! That was a very brave action to take. You're on your way to being a full-fledged intuitive eater!

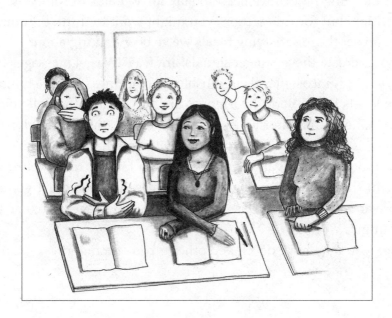

chapter 5

Do You Hear Your Stomach Growling?

On weekends, Jessica uses the clock to decide when to eat. If it's noon, it's time for lunch, and if it's six, it's time for dinner, but these rigid time rules have nothing to do with her hunger signals. Jessica said, "When I let the clock rule when I eat, sometimes I'm not hungry enough and sometimes I'm so hungry that I can't get the food in my mouth fast enough. When this happens, I don't really enjoy eating."

In this chapter, you'll explore the next Intuitive Eating principle, Honor Your Hunger. You're about to learn about different kinds of hunger and how to identify hunger, and you'll discover how great it feels when you see that food tastes even better when you're comfortably hungry!

When you were an infant, the only reason you ate was because you were hungry. Plain and simple. You felt a pang in your stomach, which probably hurt a bit, and you cried for milk. This is *physical hunger*—the purest form of hunger. And if the person who was feeding you was tuned in to your signal, you were given the gift of trust—trust in your body's signals and trust that your physical needs would be met.

Physical hunger is pretty basic. Our bodies give us signals so that we remember to eat, in order to get all the building blocks we need to stay alive. Later in the book, you'll learn about the specifics of nutrition, but for this section, you might want to think of hunger as a wonderful signal, so that you can eat those satisfying meals we've been talking about.

How do our bodies create these hunger signals, anyway? We get messages from the hypothalamus in the brain, sugar (glucose) levels in our blood, emptiness in the stomach and intestines, and some hormone levels in the body. (Hormones are messengers that tell your cells and tissues to take some action.) One of these hormones is called ghrelin (think "growl"), which is produced mainly in your gut. It is increased when you don't get enough sleep, if you've been dieting and not getting enough food (semistarvation), or are under a lot of stress. Neuropeptide Y (NPY) is a neurotransmitter in the hypothalamus, which is released if you don't get enough calories or carbohydrates (more about carbs in the last chapter). These messages all come together to let you know that you're hungry.

As you got older, you may have developed other types of hunger:

- Taste hunger

- Emotional hunger

- Experience-sharing hunger

- Energy-seeking hunger

These hungers may not be driven by physical hunger, but they all matter in our relationship with food and eating. We'll talk about all of them in this chapter, starting with physical hunger.

activity 32 ✱ getting in touch with physical hunger: signals

for you to know

If you've been dieting for a while or eating according to the clock, as Jessica did, you may have been ignoring your biological hunger signals. Or, if you're sick or filled with an emotion like anxiety, your hunger cues can be masked. In these cases, you'll have to use the logical part of your brain to tell you to eat anyway. You'll still need nourishment, even though you may not be feeling it.

The very best way to get reliable hunger signals throughout the day is to start your day with a hearty, balanced breakfast. This means having some protein, like eggs or yogurt, some carbs, like toast or cereal, and some fat, like butter or avocado on your toast or peanut butter on your oatmeal.

for you to do

There are many physical hunger signals we can feel. Put a check next to the signals you have noticed throughout the day:

☐ Stomach growling ☐ Stomach rumbling

☐ Stomach gnawing ☐ Gnawing in the throat or esophagus

When you've waited too long to eat and your blood sugar has dropped too low, the brain sends out a message that the need to eat is becoming urgent. Put a check next to the signals you've noticed when you've let your need for food go too long:

☐ Headache ☐ Light-headedness

☐ Difficulty focusing ☐ Low energy

☐ Moodiness ☐ Stomach pain

☐ Lack of concentration

In the past, how have you decided that it's time for you to eat? (Mark as many as you have experienced.)

☐ The clock told me to eat. ☐ I wanted comfort or distraction from my feelings.

☐ I felt one or more of the hunger signals listed above. ☐ Other: _____

☐ The food looked good.

Is it a rare experience for you to notice your physical hunger signals? _____

If you've felt any of the hunger signals listed above, which have you felt most often? List them here:

_____

_____

_____

_____

_____

If you don't notice hunger because you're sick or anxious, do you usually eat anyway to nourish your body?

_____

activity 33 ✳ getting in touch with physical hunger: rating your signals

for you to know

Sometimes, people don't know where to begin to get in touch with their physical hunger. Thinking about hunger and fullness in terms of a scale can help you identify the level of hunger you may be feeling. Your goal as an intuitive eater is to listen to your hunger signals and allow them to alert you that it's time to eat. If you are mostly doing this, then you've got this part down pat. If you are mostly eating for nonphysical types of hunger (like emotional hunger or taste hunger), your next job will be to practice identifying hunger signals.

for you to do

This scale will help you match your feelings of hunger with a number. We'll be using this same scale when we get to the Fullness chapter.

	Rating	Feelings of hunger and fullness
Overhungry	0	Painfully hungry. This is primal hunger. It's very intense and can actually hurt.
Overhungry	1	Ravenous and irritable. An urgent need to eat.
Overhungry	2	Extremely hungry. Intense need to find some food.
Natural Eating Range	3	Fully hungry and ready to eat.
Natural Eating Range	4	Mildly hungry, beginning to notice hunger.
Natural Eating Range	5	Neutral. Neither hungry nor full.
Natural Eating Range	6	Starting to feel satisfied.
Natural Eating Range	7	Comfortable fullness, feeling completely satisfied and content—a sign to stop.
Overfull	8	Beginning to feel a little too full. Beyond physically needing food.
Overfull	9	Extremely full and uncomfortable—everything feels tight.
Overfull	10	Stuffed and in pain. Maybe even nauseated.

The middle of the scale is 5. This is a neutral place, where you're not noticing any hunger or fullness. You're probably not even thinking of food. The natural eating range is from 3 to 4. Aiming for this range will give you the most eating satisfaction. As the numbers get smaller, your hunger will intensify until you're ravenous, and, at a 0, you'll probably feel as if you're starving. This is called primal hunger, and your tank is completely empty. And, actually, your brain senses that too and is likely to trigger overeating.

The next time you notice a hunger signal, look at the descriptions rated 0 to 4 on the Hunger/Fullness scale, and note which number matches it.

Describe your hunger signal—where do you feel it, and how does it feel?

_____

_____

Which number matches it? _____

Use the hunger part of the Hunger/Fullness scale to start guiding you to find the amount of hunger that will give you the most satisfaction, while preventing getting overfull.

activity 34 ✳ testing out taste hunger

for you to know

You might be thinking that you should be eating only when you feel a moderate signal of hunger. But what happens when you're not really hungry but have a craving for a particular taste or food? Maybe something crunchy and salty. Or maybe you see a plate of freshly baked cookies, and they look like they would taste great. People often say, "I wasn't really hungry, but I just felt like having …" These are examples of taste hunger.

Intuitive eaters are not perfect eaters. They don't always eat when they're at just the right hunger level. You're human; food is delicious, and sometimes you just want to eat something, simply for the taste of it. Don't beat yourself up when this happens.

for you to do

Throughout the coming week, keep track of the times you want to eat something just for the taste, even if you're not hungry. You can find a blank chart below and online at http://www.newhar binger.com/41443.

Day	Taste hunger foods

Here's how another teen, Tom, filled out the chart:

Day	Taste hunger foods
Monday	Half a bagel that Michael gave me at breaktime
Tuesday	Nothing
Wednesday	Nothing
Thursday	Fresh-baked cookie after school that Mom made
Friday	Nothing
Saturday	Went out for ice cream with my brother
Sunday	Candy bar at the movies

How many times did you eat something just for the taste? _____

If you notice that you're eating just because something tastes good multiple times a day, it may be that you want food for some other reason than just taste. One reason may be that you haven't fully made peace with food but grab it when it's offered, even if you're not hungry. If that's true, reread Chapter 3—Your License to Eat What You Like.

activity 35 ✳ emotional hunger

for you to know

Let's face it—food is wonderful! In fact, we spent a whole chapter on finding the ways to get the most satisfaction and pleasure out of eating. And pleasure is definitely a feeling. To say that we want to eliminate all emotional eating would mean that we would treat food simply as fuel and lose all the joy of eating. That is definitely not the goal of Intuitive Eating! In fact, if you could feel pleasure every time you ate, it would be a true gift.

But what if the emotions you're feeling actually lead you to seek food because you need comfort or want to escape feelings? If you're eating when your body doesn't need food, and it's not an occasional experience of taste hunger, then it's likely that what you're feeling is emotional hunger.

for you to do

When you filled out the chart on taste hunger, did you notice that you're eating frequently without being hungry? If you did, use the chart below to see whether emotions might be leading you to eat. For example, maybe you wanted some cookies when you felt anxious while studying for a test. Or maybe you were bored and made yourself a sandwich.

Foods eaten when not hungry	What were you feeling before you ate?

Was there one feeling that you frequently felt before eating when you weren't hungry? Perhaps it was boredom, anxiety, sadness, loneliness—or something else? In the lines below, write about what you discovered. Later in the book, you'll be learning some tools that will help you deal with these feelings.

_____

_____

_____

_____

_____

activity 36 ✱ experience-sharing hunger

for you to know

I bet you sometimes get together with your friends to go out for pizza, or go to the movies and buy popcorn and candy. That's a normal part of being a teen. But what happens if you're not hungry at those times? You definitely wouldn't want to avoid these fun, social times just because you're not at a 3 or a 4 on the hunger scale! Or sometimes you might go out to eat because of FOMO ("fear of missing out") when you're not hungry and you'd really rather stay home and finish homework or watch a movie. Being an intuitive eater means that you eat when you're physically hungry, for the most part!

for you to do

Just like eating occasionally for taste hunger, there will be times when you just want to share the experience of eating with your friends or family. Or, maybe it's the opposite, and you avoid eating with others. Answering these questions can help you evaluate this type of eating:

	Yes	No
Do I say no to going out with my friends because I'm afraid I'll eat when I'm not hungry?		
Do I eat in my room instead of eating with my family?		
Do I go out with friends but order only something to drink instead of eating with them?		
Do I eat more with friends than I do by myself or with family?		
Do I make plans with friends in order to eat foods that I don't eat at home?		
Do I say yes to going out to eat with friends just because I don't want to miss out?		
Do I pay attention to my hunger when I'm out with friends?		

The answers to the questions above will give you a lot to think about. For example, when Jessica took this quiz, she found that her rule about eating by the clock interfered with her social life. Sometimes she wouldn't go out because her friends were eating too early or too late.

On the lines below, write about what you discovered. Perhaps you've found that you have some of the same thoughts as Jessica or that you're trying to eat at a perfect hunger level and avoid social situations because you're afraid of "blowing it." That's actually a sign that you still might be in diet mentality. Or maybe you've found that you eat certain foods only when you're out with friends. That might be a hint that you live in a home where your family hasn't made peace with food. Or maybe you're not in touch with what you really need or want to be doing and go out to eat with friends even if you'd rather not, because of FOMO. What do you think about your experience-sharing hunger? Has it revealed anything that you hadn't thought about before?

_____

_____

_____

_____

_____

more to do

Write down some of the things you discovered that aren't working for you and what changes you'd like to make. Here's an example:

Problem situation: I'm avoiding social situations because I'm afraid I'll eat foods I don't think I should have.

Change you'd like to make: I'll work harder at making full peace with foods, so I can enjoy eating with friends.

Your turn:

Problem situation: _____

_____

Change you'd like to make: _____

_____

Problem situation: _____

_____

Change you'd like to make: _____

_____

Problem situation: _____

_____

Change you'd like to make: _____

_____

activity 37 ✳ energy-seeking hunger

for you to know

My hunch is that you're getting to bed very late and have to get up very early to get to school. That seems to be what happens to most teens these days. You're probably up late because you have activities after school and a lot of homework that needs to get done. You may need to connect with your friends on social media, or you're wrapped up in books or video games. Whatever the reason, it's likely that you're often feeling very tired.

Many people think that eating something when they're tired will give them more energy. This is called energy-seeking hunger. The truth is, food doesn't actually give you this kind of energy. In fact, eating when you're tired and not hungry can make you drowsy.

for you to do

Become aware of when you're experiencing energy-seeking hunger. List the times during the week when you feel tired and think that food will give you energy. Also note whether you were hungry, and write down what foods you ate. Then notice how you feel after you've eaten.

Times of feeling tired and thinking food will give you energy	Were you also hungry?	What foods did you eat?	How did you feel after eating?

If you found that you weren't actually hungry but ate several times this week because you thought it would give you energy, then, what you really need is sleep and not more food.

Becoming an intuitive eater means that you know what you need and what you feel, and you work toward getting these needs met.

If you're willing to get more sleep, write about how you can make that happen.

_____

_____

_____

_____

_____

_____

activity 38 ✳ setups for negative outcomes

for you to know

In this chapter, you've learned to pay attention to your hunger signals and to figure out when you're physically hungry and when you're "hungry" for other reasons. Your best chance of eating mainly for physical hunger is to be sure to get enough of the foods you like throughout the day. It's equally important to identify and fix any setups for negative outcomes you might still hold.

for you to do

Match the problematic setups with their outcomes by drawing a line between each. (There can be more than one outcome.)

Setup	Outcome
Waiting too long to eat	Eating excessive amounts of food you crave
Not eating balanced meals	Gulping down food
Not eating breakfast	Getting overfull
Not making peace with food	Eating foods you don't necessarily want
Not eating enough at meals	Feeling deprived
Not having sufficient coping mechanisms to deal with emotions	Eating when you're not hungry
Not getting enough sleep	Comforting yourself with food
Not paying attention to hunger signals	Avoiding feelings by eating when not hungry
Mainly hanging out with your friends during eating times	Getting hungry again too soon after eating
Not staying present when eating	Falling into primal hunger and eating too much

What did you discover when you matched up the setups and their outcomes?

_____

_____

_____

_____

_____

more to do

Name the changes you can make to be sure that you eat primarily for physical hunger, so you don't find yourself having some of the negative outcomes above. Maybe you could start eating breakfast, even if you have to take it to school with you. Or maybe you need to keep working on making peace with food or staying present when eating.

_____

_____

_____

_____

_____

chapter 6

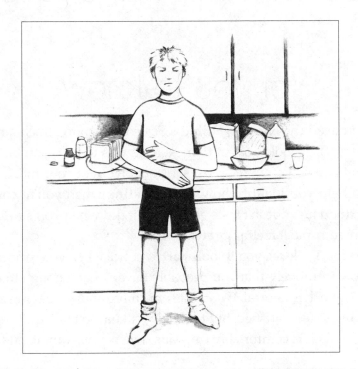

Full and Comfortable

In the last chapter, we talked about how hunger is a physical sensation that can sometimes be confusing. Its opposite, fullness, can also be misunderstood. What does fullness mean? How full is full enough but not too much? Imagine that your stomach is a balloon. You can blow a little air into it, and it will stay pretty small, or you can blow and blow until it's ready to pop. That's kind of like what your stomach can do, but, of course it's food and liquid that are going in, and maybe even a little air, if you eat or drink too fast.

Daniel loved to eat but often ate until his stomach hurt. He told me, "I love food so much that sometimes I just eat and eat until I feel like my stomach could burst. I thought I did this just because I loved food, but there must be other reasons that I have a hard time stopping."

The next Intuitive Eating principle is called Feel Your Fullness. In this chapter, you'll learn how to identify fullness, ways to find the right fullness level for you, and why you may be having a hard time noticing when you're full. Finally, you'll discover that food is actually more enjoyable when you eat to comfortable fullness. You may end up feeling a little sad that you have to stop, but I'm sure you'll decide that it's worth it.

activity 39 ✱ what fullness feels like

for you to know

In the last chapter, you used the Hunger/Fullness Scale to learn to attach a number to your level of hunger before eating. The whole goal of that exercise was to help you begin eating with comfortable hunger, so that you could get the most satisfaction out of your meal. In this chapter, we'll use the same scale to help you identify how to stop eating when you're comfortably full. Once you're past this point, food just doesn't taste as good as it did when you started, and you're at risk of walking away from your meal feeling pretty awful.

If you begin eating at a 3–4 level, you'll soon start to notice when you're not really feeling hunger anymore, but you know intuitively that you probably haven't had enough to eat. When you get to this point, you're at a 5, which is neutral. If you eat some more and are paying attention, you'll get to a 6, where you're starting to feel satisfied, but probably still haven't had quite enough. Eating a little more brings you to a 7, which is comfortably full—just where you want to end your meal.

	Rating	Feelings of hunger and fullness
Overhungry	0	Painfully hungry. This is primal hunger. It's very intense and can actually hurt.
	1	Ravenous and irritable. An urgent need to eat.
	2	Extremely hungry. Intense need to find some food.
Natural Eating Range	3	Fully hungry and ready to eat.
	4	Mildly hungry, beginning to notice hunger.
	5	Neutral. Neither hungry nor full.
	6	Starting to feel satisfied.
	7	Comfortable fullness, feeling completely satisfied and content—a sign to stop.
Overfull	8	Beginning to feel a little too full. Beyond physically needing food.
	9	Extremely full and uncomfortable—everything feels tight.
	10	Stuffed and in pain. Maybe even nauseated.

for you to do

In order to figure out the right fullness level for you, fill out the chart below for at least three days. You can find this chart at http://www.newharbinger.com/41443. What and how much you eat will determine how long your fullness lasts and when you start to feel hungry again. The first row of the chart comes from Daniel's experience.

Time you ate	What you ate and about how much	Fullness number when you stopped (0–10)	How many hours before you got hungry again
Noon	Four pieces of pizza and two cookies	9	6

What did you notice about how long your meals lasted you? For example, if you ate only a salad, did you stop at a comfortable fullness (7 on the chart), but get hungry again in two hours? Same goes for snacks—popcorn or an apple will tide you over for only a short time. Or did you finish all of a pretty filling meal and not get hungry again for five hours, or a rich snack like a big candy bar and not be hungry for dinner? Some foods like salad, which is filled with fiber and water, or popcorn that has a lot of air and fiber can give you an artificial sense of fullness, so don't be surprised if you got hungry again quickly.

Write about what you discovered:

_____

_____

_____

_____

    Do this exercise as many times as you need until you're able to find the foods in a meal that will give you just the right comfortable fullness and will last you about three to four hours. But remember, you have the license to eat whatever you like. If you choose to eat foods that don't last you very long or that last longer than expected, that's cool too. There's no perfect fullness level, just the one that works for you at any given time.

activity 40 ✱ learning to identify fullness: staying present

for you to know

Feeling comfortably full can be a wonderful, satisfying feeling after you've had a delicious meal. But for some people, it's hard to identify fullness, and you might mismatch your fullness number to your actual fullness. Maybe you've become so used to feeling your "balloon" stretched to the max that you think you're comfortably full when you're actually overfull. Or maybe you think you're full, but you haven't really had enough to eat.

Here are some ways to begin identifying the right level of fullness for you:

- Stay present when eating.

- Eat slowly.

- Eat every few hours, so you don't go into primal hunger.

- Start eating when you're comfortably hungry.

- Pay attention to why you started eating.

There's one more point to consider in identifying fullness, and it has to do with what you've learned in your family about when to finish your meal: be aware of any family rules about finishing your plate.

Each of the next six activities (starting with this one) will explore one of these points. We start with the idea of staying present, because it's actually the key to putting all the Intuitive Eating principles into action.

for you to do

Staying present means that you're not multitasking and paying attention to other things while eating. When people do that, they often get distracted from noticing if the food is satisfying their taste buds and when they're getting comfortably full. In the chart below, mark some of the activities you might do while eating. On a scale of 1–3, note how much each distracts you. (1 equals not at all, 2 means it distracts you a bit, and 3 means you're completely distracted.) Daniel put a check by watching TV, surfing the internet, and texting. He gave all of these activities a 3 because they completely distracted him from noticing when he got full.

Activities while eating	✓	How much does this activity distract you from your meal? (Scale of 1–3)
Texting		
Watching TV		
Doing homework		
Surfing the internet		
Talking on the phone		
Checking out social media		
Playing a video game		
Reading a book		
Glancing at a magazine		
Eating with the family		
Eating with friends		
Driving		
Walking		
Other: _____		
Other: _____		

Which activities were the most distracting?

_____

_____

_____

_____

Pick one of these distracting activities that you're willing to change, and after you've changed it, pay attention to whether you were able to notice when you became comfortably full. Write about it here:

_____

_____

_____

_____

activity 41 ✳ learning to identify fullness: eating slowly

for you to know

In the chapter Savor and Be Satisfied, eating slowly was one of the tips for being able to notice satisfaction. Well, it will also give you the best chance of finding comfortable fullness. Here are three things that happen when you eat slowly:

- Your body releases more fullness hormones that signal the brain that you're full and can stop eating. One of these is called leptin. (Note: If you've been undereating and have lost weight, your leptin levels are reduced—one of the reasons diets end up making you feel hungrier and crave more food.)

- You're able to recognize the signals these hormones give you.

- You're also able to notice the point at which food doesn't taste as good as it did when you started. This is called the *last-bite threshold*, and it shows up at just about the same time that you're comfortably full.

for you to do

For this exercise, find a time when you're hungry and aren't distracted. You might want to do this when you're alone and able to focus on the exercise. Begin your meal when you're at a hunger level of about 3—not ravenous, but fully ready to eat. (See the Hunger/Fullness Scale at the beginning of this chapter.)

What foods did you pick for your meal?

_____

_____

_____

Begin eating, and chew your food, rather than gulping it down.

As you eat, put your fork (or sandwich) down after each bite.

Swallow before you take the next bite. (Lots of people put the next bite in their mouths while they're still chewing!)

Take a time-out about two-thirds through your meal. What are you feeling now? Are you at a neutral point, or do you notice any fullness creeping in?

_____

_____

Do you think you still need a few more bites? _____

As fullness shows up, what do you notice about how your food tastes? _____

At this point, fullness will match up with less enjoyment, and you've found the last-bite threshold. It's probably the time when you're ready to stop eating. Some people feel sad when they realize that their body is full, and they need to stop. In the next chapter, we'll explore the feelings that can come up when this happens.

activity 42 ✱ learning to identify fullness: avoiding primal hunger

for you to know

In the last chapter, you learned that when you're in primal hunger, you feel completely ravenous and feel as if there won't be enough food to fill you. And, boy, do you ever fill yourself! You might have a hard time stopping. You want to avoid this predicament as much as you can. If you start eating with primal hunger, you're likely to end feeling miserably full. The best way to solve this problem is to:

- Start with a balanced breakfast, as we talked about in the last chapter.

- Start eating when you're comfortably hungry (about a 3 or 4), not ravenous.

- Eat about every three to four hours.

- Eat balanced meals and snacks.

for you to do

If your meals are balanced, it will be easier to notice when you're becoming comfortably full. Balanced meals include protein, fat, carbohydrate, and fiber. Here are some examples of balanced lunches:

- Peanut butter and jelly sandwich, a few raw carrots, a handful of chips, a glass of milk, and an apple

- A couple of sushi rolls, some edamame, and an orange

- Salad with chicken, avocado, shredded cheese, a few crackers or a couple of bread rolls, and some grapes

111

Write down some balanced lunches that you'd enjoy:

_____

_____

_____

_____

Examples of balanced dinners:

- A couple of enchiladas with cheese, some rice and beans

- Hamburger, some fries, and a small salad

- Two or three pieces of pizza and some carrots and celery

Your turn for some ideas of balanced dinners:

_____

_____

_____

_____

And now, how about some balanced snacks that could keep you going for an hour or two until your next meal?

- Hummus and carrots

- String cheese and crackers

- Peanut or almond butter and an apple

- Nuts and grapes

- Trail mix

What are your favorite snacks?

_____

_____

_____

_____

Choosing foods you typically select, track your eating for one day, including the times of eating, how many hours since you last ate, the foods eaten, your hunger level at the beginning of eating, and your fullness level when you're done:

Time of meal	Hours since last meal	Foods eaten	Hunger level at start	Fullness level at end

When you evaluate your chart, do you notice any trends? For example, are you waiting too long between meals and getting overhungry, or are you eating so often that you don't get a chance to feel hungry? Are your meals balanced? Are you eating a lot of "air" food, like popcorn?

_____

_____

_____

_____

more to do

Using what you learned after tracking a typical eating day, make some changes to include more balance in your meals. You might also try foods that have more substance and less air. Use the chart at http://www.newharbinger.com/41443 again to see what effect these changes make.

What have you learned about noticing fullness by making these changes?

_____

_____

_____

_____

activity 43 ✱ learning to identify fullness: starting to eat when you're comfortably hungry

for you to know

I absolutely love eating—if I begin to eat when I feel some moderate hunger. We've already talked about starting at this point in order to get the most satisfaction from your meal. But, to me, there's another important advantage to feeling this sense of hunger at the beginning of your meal. If you don't feel hunger when you start, you have no reference point to detect those first signs of fullness. The natural path of eating goes from moderate hunger (3–4), moving on to neutral (5—no sense of hunger or fullness), and stopping when you're comfortably full and satisfied (6–7). Just like there's day and night, there's hunger and fullness. It's all about contrast!

for you to do

This exercise takes true mindfulness from beginning to end. Do it when you're in a quiet place and are able to be fully present with your meal.

Begin eating with moderate hunger, and notice if you can feel those first signs of comfortable fullness creeping in. You may need a few more bites after that to reach the last-bite threshold. Then end your meal and write about your experience. Did you notice the contrast between hunger and fullness? Did starting when you were moderately hungry make it easier to recognize your stopping point?

_____

_____

_____

_____

activity 44 ✳ learning to identify fullness: paying attention to why you start eating

for you to know

In an ideal world of intuitive eating, you would usually begin each eating experience simply because you were hungry. But as you learned in the last chapter, there are many kinds of hunger. Review these so that you have them fresh in your mind to help you determine your reason for eating. Is it hunger or emotions or simply taste? And why is this important? Well, your best chance of satisfying your tongue and your body has to do with this whole hunger and fullness thing.

You may be getting tired of hearing me talk about satisfaction, but I'm willing to take that risk, because I think it's the gift of intuitive eating. Learning to stop eating when you're comfortably full is a skill that takes lots of practice, but the reward is so worth the task. That reward is feeling comfortable and satisfied.

for you to do

Understanding what's behind your decision to start eating will help you figure out whether that reason will bring you the end result you want.

Plan to feel your fullness for the majority of your meals for the next two days. You can use the chart below, or at http://www.newharbinger.com/41443. To help you practice, ask yourself why you're about to eat, each time you begin. Is it for hunger (comfortable or primal)? Mainly taste? Emotions? Experience sharing? Energy seeking?

Daniel did this exercise to figure out the reasons why he regularly ate until his stomach hurt. The first row of the chart shows what he discovered for one meal.

Meal	Why are you about to eat?	Were you able to notice comfortable fullness?
Lunch	I'm ravenously hungry because I haven't eaten anything all day.	Not really, because I inhaled the food.

Daniel discovered that starting to eat when he was in primal hunger was one of the reasons he frequently overate. You'll find that you'll more often be able to notice comfortable fullness if you begin eating for comfortable hunger rather than for primal hunger, taste hunger, or any of the other hungers. The further you get on the path to noticing your fullness, the easier it will be to stop eating at the best fullness level for you.

After you've practiced the last five exercises for a while, come back to answer these questions:

Are you finding that you're becoming an expert at identifying comfortable fullness? How does this feel for you?

_____

_____

_____

_____

activity 45 ✳ learning to identify fullness: navigating family rules

for you to know

In the chapter that gave you the license to eat what you like, you did a lot of work hunting down your food rules and where they came from. One rule that might have come from your family is "Clean your plate before you leave the table." If this is true for you, you'll need to use your skills at banishing the Food Police to wipe it out of your brain.

for you to do

If you hold this rule, it's likely that it came from your family. To help you see if it's "ruling" you, put a check next to the statements that describe you:

☐ I finish everything on my plate most of the time.

☐ If I'm eating something that comes in a package, I finish the whole package.

☐ I always finish a whole apple, no matter how big it is.

☐ I rarely got enough food when I was growing up.

☐ If I'm eating a sandwich, I make sure to finish both halves.

☐ I think it's wasteful to leave any food on my plate.

☐ At a buffet, I go back several times to get more food.

☐ I have to finish all my food before I can have dessert.

☐ I feel guilty if I don't finish my food.

☐ It doesn't matter how full I am—I want it all!

How many checks do you have? _____

Even one check might mean that you were taught to clean your plate when you were younger. If you discovered that you're still following your family's rule about cleaning your plate, pay attention to how this rule operates in your family. Here are some red flags to look for:

• The food is plated before you arrive at the table. No one is consulted about their hunger and how much food they need.

• When you put your fork down and don't move to pick it up even though there's still food on your plate, you're told that you haven't eaten enough.

• Everyone stays at the table until all the food on the plates is gone.

more to do

Letting go of this rule brings you closer to being an intuitive eater. Here are some strategies to help you break it and eat intuitively:

- Let the person who cooked the meal know that it was delicious and that you appreciate it.

- When you notice that you're comfortably full, ask if you can save the rest of your food to eat if you get hungry later, or to eat the next day.

- Let your family know that when you eat more than your body needs, you end up feeling stuffed, and you don't want to be uncomfortable.

- If you're forced to keep eating until you finish everything, comfort yourself by knowing that you'll be able to honor your fullness when you're not eating at home.

Write about how you plan to use these strategies and what you hope the outcome will be.

_____

_____

_____

_____

_____

even more to do

Take the quiz at http://www.newharbinger.com/41443 to see if you're no longer trapped by the "clean the plate rule" (or maybe never were).

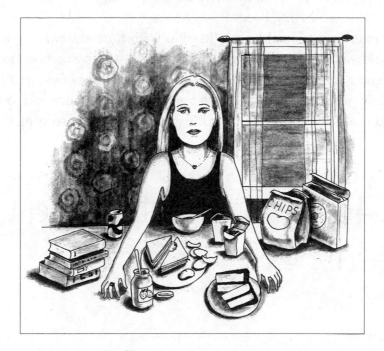

chapter 7

Is Food Your Frenemy?

Have you ever had a friend who can be comforting one day and make you feel terrible the next? If you have, you probably realize how confusing it is for the same person to be both positive and negative in your life. We call this kind of person a frenemy, and food can also play this very role.

Melissa had a similar problem to Daniel's, but for different reasons. She had tears in her eyes when she told me, "I'm just so frustrated. I love food so much and look forward to eating when I'm hungry, but sometimes I keep on eating after I'm full and end up hating the food and myself. Food has become my enemy. I really need help to understand why I do this. I want to be an intuitive eater, and I want food to be my friend, not my enemy. Please help me!"

In this chapter you'll find tools that helped Melissa (and will help you, too) make food a loving part of life, instead of a frenemy. The Intuitive Eating principle this chapter centers on is Cope with Your Emotions Without Using Food.

Developing an emotionally healthy relationship with food starts with doing some work on your own emotional health, including practicing self-care, feeling compassion rather than judgment for yourself (and all your emotions, even the uncomfortable ones), and reminding yourself that food can not only give you physical health but also offer pleasure and satisfaction when you eat intuitively. Food is about supporting your life, not running it or ruining it.

activity 46 ✳ understanding why people eat

for you to know

Food can serve many purposes in our lives. Here are some of them:

- *Nourishment*—duh! We all know that we need food to take care of our hunger, give us energy, help us heal wounds, make our bones stronger, and grow taller, among other reasons.

- *Pleasure*—Eating a great meal when we're hungry can be one of the most pleasurable and satisfying experiences of life. In fact, we spent a whole chapter on this goal.

- *Comfort*—Food just seems to have the magical power sometimes to make us feel better when we're upset. We often learn this as babies or toddlers when we fall down or go to the doctor, and we're given some ice cream or a lollipop to stop us from crying.

- *Procrastination*—When we really don't feel like doing our work, we sometimes run into the kitchen to find something to eat. The problem is, we still have to do the work and end up feeling rushed and stressed.

- *Distraction*—Some of us use food when we're bored or to distract ourselves from tough feelings. There's a problem here, too, since the feeling isn't really going to go away until you deal with it, so this is actually another form of procrastination.

- *Numbing*—Sometimes the emotions that bubble up in us seem so difficult that we end up wanting to eat and eat, or perhaps avoid eating to numb us from feeling anything. Either way, the feelings end up becoming even bigger and harder to deal with, and on top of it, your body ends up hurting from being too full or from feeling starved.

- *Punishment*—People who are feeling really bad about themselves can use food as a way to hurt themselves. If this is something you do, it's important that you talk to someone about your distress. If you can't talk to your parents, you might feel safe with a teacher, school counselor, a friend's parent, religious leader, or psychotherapist. Hurting yourself is not an option!

for you to do

Do you have a hunch about the main reasons why you eat? Number these reasons from one to seven, with one being the reason you most often eat and seven being the least. If you experience two or more equally, you can give them the same number.

_____ Nourishment

_____ Pleasure

_____ Comfort

_____ Procrastination

_____ Distraction

_____ Numbing

_____ Punishment

Which two reason(s) were at the top of your list?

_____

_____

Which two were at the bottom?

_____

_____

If at the top of your list you named reasons other than nourishment and pleasure, the rest of this chapter will help you turn your list upside down!

activity 47 ✳ practicing compassion

for you to know

Life can bring us difficult emotions and situations. Sometimes we haven't learned enough healthy coping skills to deal with these, so we find whatever is available in the moment to get us through. Eating or restricting food are often the most immediate ways we attempt to take care of ourselves. Rather than beating yourself up for this, be compassionate toward yourself, and understand that it was the best you could do at the time.

The quality of compassion includes sensitivity and feelings toward others, patience and wisdom, kindness, warmth, care, and a desire to relieve suffering. You may be very skilled at showing compassion to others, but how compassionate are you toward yourself?

Without compassion, life can feel insurmountable, and it's possible that you'll turn toward or away from food for comfort, as a hiding place, or as a way to punish yourself.

for you to do

In the chart that follows, you'll find some negative statements that people often make about themselves. Mark any that sound familiar to you. On a scale of 1–5, with 1 showing the least compassion and 5 the most, rate how compassionate you feel toward yourself around these statements. Add any similar statements of your own, and rate your self-compassion. At the top of the chart, you'll find an example from Melissa's chart.

Statement	Sound familiar?	Self-compassion rating (1–5)
When I'm anxious about schoolwork, I run to food.	✓	3
I seem to overeat all the time.		
I can't fit into some of my clothes.		
I've spent my life hating myself.		
I keep failing on diets.		
I eat when I'm not hungry.		
I use food to soothe myself when I'm sad.		
I won't let myself eat what I want.		
I don't eat enough when I'm anxious.		
I'm a couch potato—I hardly ever move.		
I have a hard time with school.		
I don't think people like me.		

Statement	Sound familiar?	Self-compassion rating (1–5)

more to do

Choose a few of the statements above for which you were less compassionate. Practice positive self-talk—speaking to yourself in kind words—such as "I was going through a rough time and am glad I had food to comfort me." Here's an example of how Melissa began to show more compassion toward herself for running to food when she was anxious about school:

Negative self-talk—*What's wrong with me? I'm always running to food when I'm super stressed.*

Positive self-talk—*There's so much pressure to get all my homework done and go to soccer practice and stay in touch with my friends. I understand that food comforts me when I'm so overwhelmed. It's been the best I could do, and now I'm working on new coping skills that will help me not use food to calm myself.*

Write several sentences that show a shift from your own negative self-talk to positive self-talk.

Negative self-talk _____

_____

Positive self-talk _____

_____

_____

Negative self-talk _____

_____

Positive self-talk _____

_____

_____

Negative self-talk _____

_____

Positive self-talk _____

_____

_____

_____

activity 48 ✱ practicing gratitude

for you to know

Another important tool to help you manage life's difficulties is gratitude. People often spend lots of time focused on what others have that they don't have and on feeling the despair of their deprivation. If you can flip this focus and look for the things in your life that you appreciate, you'll find that your mood will switch, and your need to use eating as a way to cope will shrink away.

for you to do

In the chart that follows, you'll find some things to put on a gratitude list. Mark the ones that fit for you and then add any others:

I am grateful for:	Yes or No
My family	
My friends	
My pets	
My significant other	
My health	
My education	

My artistic or musical talent	
My athletic ability	
The way I can dance	
My spirituality	

more to do

Tomorrow morning, make a gratitude list in your mind or write it in your phone or your notebook. Every time you're feeling down, look at your list. At the end of the day, use the space below to write about how doing this made you feel.

_____

_____

_____

_____

_____

_____

even more to do

Make a gratitude list every day for two weeks (you can download a copy at http://www.newharbinger.com/41443). Then go back and do activity 47 again. Notice any difference?

activity 49 ✳ exploring your range of emotions

for you to know

Once you've become more self-compassionate and recognize that your relationship with food is actually serving you as a coping mechanism, you're ready to start figuring out your emotions and finding healthy coping mechanisms to deal with them.

Emotions can range from very positive ones, such as joy or excitement, to very painful ones, like anxiety and fear. Here are some of the most common emotions people feel:

pleasure	fear
joy	anxiety
excitement	sadness
boredom	loneliness
disappointment	shame
frustration	guilt
anger	

for you to do

This week, keep a journal of all the emotions you notice you're feeling, how many times you feel them, and how you handle them. For example, you may have felt some anxiety or sadness and handled it by one or more of the following coping mechanisms:

- eating when you weren't hungry

- not eating enough food

- talking to someone about your feelings

- writing in a journal

- overexercising

- taking a walk

- getting started on a task you're avoiding

- taking deep breaths

- meditating

- taking things one tiny step at a time when you're overwhelmed

Use these lines to add others:

_____

_____

_____

_____

_____

_____

At the end of the week, fill in this chart to get a snapshot of your emotional range and how you handled various emotions. (Note: You might handle the same emotion differently at different times.)

Emotion	How many times you felt it	How you handled it
Pleasure		
Joy		
Excitement		
Boredom		
Disappointment		
Frustration		
Anger		
Fear		
Anxiety		
Sadness		
Loneliness		
Shame		
Guilt		
Other: _____		
Other: _____		
Other: _____		

more to do

Looking at the chart above, what were the main coping mechanisms you used to get you through these emotions? Write them here:

_____

_____

_____

_____

_____

_____

How often did you discover that food was involved in the way you coped?

Frequently _____   Sometimes _____   Rarely _____

If you find that you're frequently eating beyond your comfortable fullness, looking for food when you're not hungry, or not allowing yourself to eat when you are hungry, you may realize that food has become your frenemy. If this is true for you, remember to be compassionate with yourself and throw out any feelings of shame or guilt.

activity 50 ✳ practicing self-care

for you to know

If food has become your enemy, it's time to learn how to make it your friend again—one that gives you nourishment and satisfaction.

If you've ever gone hiking, you know that you're often given a choice of several paths. One is usually the easiest, one the hardest, and some are in between. The same goes for the different paths toward healing your emotional eating. One may be easier for some people, while another is easier for others. Easy or hard, each one builds on the others to finally help free you from emotional eating.

for you to do

Are you someone who takes very good care of yourself? Maybe you floss every day and get enough sleep most nights. If so, bravo! But sometimes it's really hard to do everything people tell you you need to do. Self-care is so important, because if you're not paying attention to your needs, you're at greater risk for looking for food as a way to care for yourself.

Are you on top of these self-care habits?

	Yes	No
Getting enough sleep five out of seven nights		
Getting enough food most days, so you have plenty of energy and can concentrate on your school work		
Keeping your body and your teeth clean		
Finding balance in your life, so that you're not focused only on school or social life		
Getting enough movement in your life, like dancing, taking walks, participating in a sport, and others		
Having people in your life to talk to when you're having problems		
Finding ways to have fun and laugh		
Exploring ways to be creative		
Wearing clothes that you like and are comfortable		

If you answered yes to at least seven of these habits, you're doing an amazing job of taking care of your needs. List any areas where you could improve your self-care, and check the first ones you'd like to work on:

_____

_____

_____

_____

_____

_____

_____

more to do

Here are some ideas about improving some of your self-care habits:

- silencing your phone and not looking at your feeds about a half hour earlier than usual each night in order to get better sleep. (Note: The light in your phone actually interferes with the quality of your sleep.)

- taking your dog for walks more often or taking a walk after breakfast on weekend mornings in order to put more movement into your life

- starting a regular chat among a few safe friends where you can vent your problems

- finding counseling help, if problems feel overwhelming

Brainstorm some ideas about how you could work on some of the habits that need focus:

_____

_____

_____

_____

_____

_____

About once a week, take a look at your list of ideas to evaluate whether you've made progress in self-care. If you have, write about how that feels and how you can add even more self-care to your life.

_____

_____

_____

_____

_____

_____

activity 51 ✳ finding balance

for you to know

Finding balance in your life is the fourth self-care habit on the list in activity 50. It's sometimes the hardest to achieve. When you put too much energy into one part of your life, you're likely neglecting other important parts. This can lead to anxiety about getting everything done, with the potential of using food to calm yourself.

for you to do

In the pie chart following, write an important part of your life in each space. Here are some examples:

school   grooming

homework   creativity

friends   sleep

dating   social media

family   spirituality

sports or movement

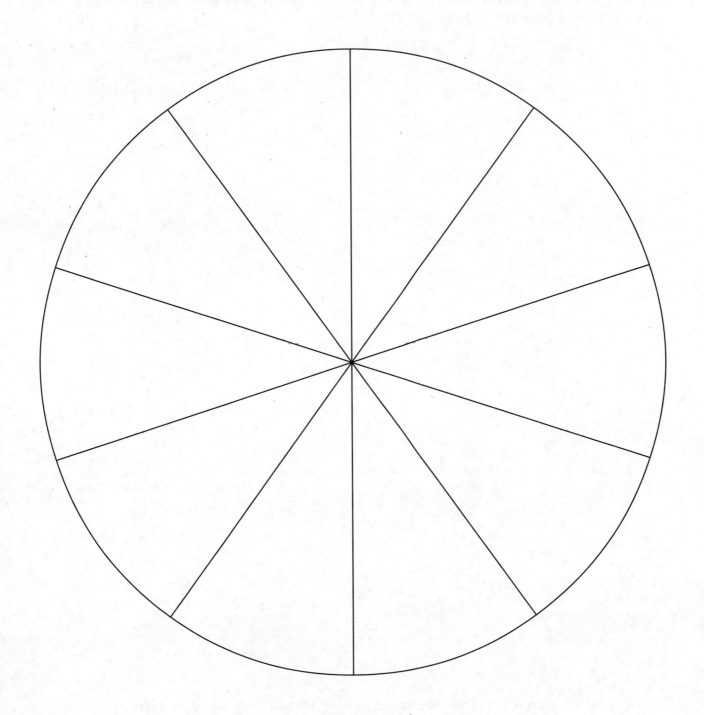

Now, draw your own circle and space out the size of each slice according to how much of your life it takes up. For example, you might have half of your pie assigned to school and smaller slices of your life in the other half.

When Melissa drew her circle, she found that her slice of sleep was very small and her slice of social media very big. She also found that she didn't even have a slice of her life dedicated to painting, which she loved. By limiting her social media time, she found time for creativity.

Does your life look balanced, or do you need to consider whether too much time is taken up in one or two areas? If so, draw as many circles as you need in your notebook and practice sizing the slices the way you would like them to look. Don't strive for even slices, because that's not realistic or even possible—just try for more balance to meet your needs.

Write about how you might expand some slices and shrink others in order to feel more balance in your life:

_____

_____

_____

_____

_____

_____

activity 52 ✳ feeling the power of nurturance

for you to know

In the last section, you thought about all the basic ways that self-care is part of your life. Nurturing yourself goes beyond these basics. Some people might call nurturance self-indulgence, but to me, that's a very judgmental way of understanding the special things that can make you feel that your needs are being met. Everyone has very deep needs for feeling special. These needs can be met by doing something nice for yourself or by asking others to nurture you.

Here are some ways to feel nurtured:

bubble baths

hot showers for aching muscles

manicures or pedicures

using oils, lotions, or colognes

asking for hugs and back rubs

reading a book for pleasure

listening to your favorite music

buying yourself a present you can afford

calling your best friend when you're upset

playing with your pet

meditating

speaking to yourself with kindness and compassion

for you to do

Some of the ways you've self-soothed in the past, especially using food, only stand in for nurturance. True nurturance involves tender and loving self-care, both physically and emotionally.

How do you presently nurture yourself? Which ways are truly nurturing for you? For example—physical comfort and care, building more connections with others, being kind to yourself.

_____

_____

_____

_____

more to do

List some other truly nurturing experiences you would like to bring into your life:

_____

_____

_____

_____

The more nurturance in your life, the less your chance of turning to food as a coping mechanism.

activity 53 ✳ building your emotional muscle: sit with difficult feelings

for you to know

Whether you're taking ballet, training for a sport, or hiking, you're not only gaining a skill but also strengthening your body's muscles. You can think about your emotional strength in the same way. This activity, and the two that follow, will help you build emotional muscle.

One of the best ways is to learn to "sit with" difficult feelings—not trying to run from them or numb them but taking care of yourself as these feelings arise and pass away. By sitting with your feelings, you will soon develop a way to tolerate difficult emotions, while strengthening your emotional muscle.

for you to do

For this exercise, you will need to have a quiet place that's comfortable and safe. You won't want to have your younger sibling bursting in to ask you to play or a parent knocking on the door, telling you to do a chore.

Can you think of a place that would work for you? For example, sitting in your car, on the beach, or a bench in a park? List any places that could become your private place:

_____

_____

_____

_____

The next time you feel a feeling that is hard to handle, go to your private place. Bring your journal, and note the time. Sit (or lie) down, and take a few deep breaths, noticing the air going in and out of your lungs. This will help calm you.

Notice how your body feels. Feel the bottoms of your feet, your hands, your back, or any other part of your body.

Focus on a flower or a tree or anything else. Notice the shape and color.

Now, look at the time again and see how many minutes you've tolerated this difficult feeling.

_____

Afterward, write about your feelings. (Some people might want to write on their phones, but it works much better if you actually write by hand in your journal. The physical act of writing by hand can help you release feelings, especially anxiety and stress.)

Do you feel any better or calmer now? _____

Breathing, grounding yourself, noticing your surroundings, and writing are powerful tools that can help you develop your emotional muscle. Do this exercise whenever feelings start to overcome you. You will notice over time that you'll be able to sit with them longer, without using food.

activity 54 ✻ building your emotional muscle: allow the sadness of saying "enough"

for you to know

Have you ever experienced that point in a meal when you're full but don't want to stop eating? When the food is delicious and you know you've had enough, it's very possible that a feeling of sadness will show up. (Sometimes it's a feeling other than sadness—we'll talk about this in the next activity.) Any time we're doing something pleasurable, it's very normal to be filled with sadness about having to stop. Whether it's the end of a vacation or a good date or a wonderful meal, it's likely you'll feel sad. Acknowledging that feeling will help you get through the few moments it takes to pass. If you get involved in another activity, before you know it, the sadness is gone. This is another way of learning to "sit with" difficult feelings.

for you to do

The next time you're eating a yummy meal, notice how you feel when you realize you're comfortably full. If you feel sad, see if you can sit for five minutes before eating more. (Remember—there are more satisfying meals to come!) Then remove your plate or leave the table and begin another activity. Write about this experience of sadness, sitting with it, and moving on from the meal to another activity.

_____

_____

_____

_____

Try this several times over the course of a week or two. Are there any activities that work better than others to help you move beyond the sadness?

_____

_____

_____

_____

activity 55 ✳ building your emotional muscle: get to know what you feel and what you really need

for you to know

Sometimes a feeling deeper than sadness arises when you want to eat but you're not hungry, or you notice fullness during a meal but want to keep eating. To handle this feeling, the question to ask is: what do I feel, and what do I really need now?

If your body needs only a certain amount of food to feel comfortably full, but you regularly want more, it's a surefire sign of a need in your life that's begging for attention. (Note: You have a right to have needs and to have your needs met.)

Here are some of the needs people have:

- to be around others

- to feel comforted by someone

- to talk out feelings with someone safe

- to release some steam or nervous energy

- to stimulate their minds

for you to do

The next time you have a strong urge to eat when you're not hungry, ask yourself: "What am I feeling?"

_____

_____

_____

Then ask, "What do I really need?"

Name some of the things that you might actually need instead of food at this time. Put stars next to the needs that feel the strongest, or the most frequent.

_____

_____

_____

_____

_____

_____

Now brainstorm some ways to meet those needs without turning to food or food-centered behaviors. Which one would you like to try out in the next few days?

_____

_____

_____

activity 56 ✳ using helpful distraction

for you to know

Sometimes it's simply too hard to figure out a feeling or to cope with it. What a dilemma! You don't want to use food, yet you can't deal with the feeling that's coming up. This is the time to find a temporary distracting activity that doesn't involve food, until you can get some help.

Here are some activities that might work:

- watching a movie or a TV show
- hanging out with friends
- playing with your pet
- reading a good book
- scanning the internet

- listening to music
- playing an instrument
- moving your body

for you to do

Name some activities that might help distract you for a while. Think about where and when difficult feelings might arise and what you might do in that time and place to (safely!) distract yourself without involving food. Put stars next to the ones you'd like to try.

_____

_____

_____

_____

activity 57 ✳ preparing and rehearsing

for you to know

A powerful tactic for avoiding emotional eating is to prepare for and rehearse triggering situations. To prepare:

- Notice if you have any anxiety about an upcoming event and are worried about how eating will go.

- Leading up to the event, eat regularly. If you cut back, you're bound to overdo when you get there.

- If the event is far from home or will last a long time, bring snacks so you're not caught hungry with nothing to eat.

- Make plans to call or text someone if you become upset.

To rehearse:

- Imagine yourself at the event, eating enough to be satisfied but not overfull.

- See yourself coming home, feeling great that you ate enough—not too little or too much.

- Rehearse what you'll do if you become anxious or bored. Perhaps, contact someone, take a break and walk outside, breathe deeply, or something else?

for you to do

Here is an example of an event that worried Melissa:

My sister's bridal shower is in two weeks. There'll be a ton of food, and also a ton of my sister's sorority friends. I'll be the youngest one there, and they're her friends, not mine. One of her bridesmaids, Trish—I think she thinks I'm dumb, or something. I have to go, but I'm not going to enjoy it.

Think of a worrisome event coming up in your life. What's worrying about it, in particular? Write about it here:

_____

_____

_____

_____

Visualize the event from beginning to end: how do you think it will go, and how do you see yourself during each part of the event?

Melissa wrote: *I'm probably going to be bored and feel like I don't belong. There'll be lots of bowls of chips, nuts, and candy, and I'll be tempted to eat a lot to help the boredom and anxiety about not fitting in. Then there'll be lunch, which might be hard, too.*

Now describe your event in the same way:

_____

_____

_____

_____

How will you prepare and rehearse for the hard parts you foresee?

Melissa wrote: *I'll take a small plate and put some snacks on it, but not too many, because I want to have some hunger for lunch. Then I'll ask my sister if I can sit near her at lunch, so I'm more comfortable. If I'm feeling too much boredom or anxiety, I'll excuse myself for a minute and go text my best friend for support.*

Your turn:

_____

_____

_____

_____

_____

How did it go?

Melissa wrote: *Wow, by preparing and rehearsing, I got through this shower really well. Since I didn't overeat, I was able to focus on the presents being opened, and I even got to talk to one of my sister's friends, who was really nice to me. And Trish was okay too! It ended up feeling so good!*

After your worrisome event, write about how it went:

_____

_____

_____

_____

_____

Anticipation (preparation) and visualization (rehearsal) are powerful ways to overcome future emotional eating. The more you practice these skills, the more fun you'll have and the less stress you'll feel.

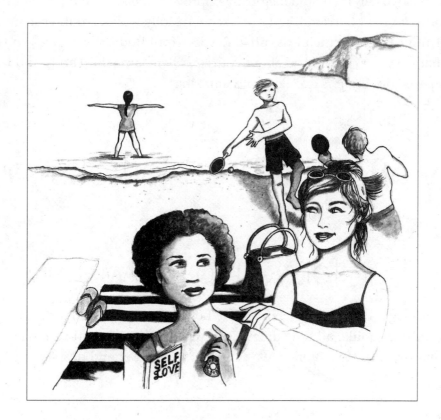

chapter 8

Your Body: Temple, Fortress, or Foe?

In the best of all worlds, we'd all be grateful for the many wonderful things our bodies can do. We'd accept that bodies come in different sizes and shapes and that all of them are worthy. We'd also accept that our bodies are genetically programmed to look the way they do—height, eye and hair color, shape, and, most importantly, weight. Unfortunately, the real world we live in can regularly make us feel bad about our bodies.

Molly feels so bad about herself that she regularly makes negative comments about her body. She once told me, "I don't think I'm smart enough or that very many people like me. I haven't liked my body for a very long time. I decided that if I could restrict my food enough, I'd finally like myself. But, guess what—it's not working. I still don't like my body, and nothing has changed in the way I feel about myself."

Molly has bought in to all the media hype that promises her that if she could only change her body, everything else in her life would magically improve. Instead of being grateful for her healthy body, kind parents, loving boyfriend, and great school, Molly walks around sad and discouraged.

The next Intuitive Eating principle is called Respect Your Body, and it gives you tools for fighting the forces that want you to feel bad about your (excellent, amazing) body and learning to love it instead (because, seriously, it *is* excellent and amazing).

activity 58 ✱ temple, fortress, or foe?

for you to know

Teens have many ways of thinking about their bodies (actually adults do too). The way you approach your body can make all the difference in whether life is mostly an interesting, exciting, pleasurable adventure—or feels more like a prison of self-hatred and despair.

for you to do

Mark any of the statements that describe your thoughts:

1. I'm proud that my body is strong enough to_____
   (for example: swim, dance, hike, do yoga, play a sport, pull my wheelchair).

2. All the other kids' bodies are better than mine.

3. My body deserves kind words.

4. Because I don't like my body, I never go to the beach or pool.

5. I love to go shopping and buy clothes I like.

6. I'll never have a significant other because my body isn't good enough.

7. I'd rather stay in my room playing video games or being on social media than hang out with other people.

8. I take really good care of my body.

9. I'm too short. *Or,* I don't like my feet. *Or,* I wish I were thinner. *Or,* I don't like my hair. *Or,* I wish I had big muscles. *Or* _____.

10. I love to take selfies with my friends.

11. I'm lucky to have the body I have.

12. My body protects me from feeling hurt.

If you marked 1, 3, 5, 8, 10 and 11, you feel your body is your temple.

If you marked 4, 7, or 12, your body may be the fortress that keeps you safe but isolated.

And, if you marked 2, 6, or 9, you unfortunately see your body as your foe.

Is your body your temple, your fortress, your foe, or some of each?

---

activity 59 ✳ unlocking the door to the fortress

for you to know

If you discovered that your body is your temple, you can celebrate your great self-care, body appreciation, and positive self-talk. Living life with gratitude for all that your body is and can do is the launching pad for a lifetime of self-love.

If you discovered that your body is your fortress, you've probably been using your negative feelings about it to protect you from taking risks.

for you to do

You used a pro and con list earlier in this book to weigh the benefits and downside of dieting. This same exercise will help you look at whether using your body as your fortress is working for you.

For example, because Molly felt so bad about her body, she stayed home from parties and other activities. The first row of the chart below shows how Molly used the list to help her weigh the outcome of her decision. You can use the rest of the chart in the same way. If your cons outweigh your pros, it's likely that your negative body thoughts are keeping you from living your fullest life.

Issue	Pros	Cons
Not going to parties because I'm embarrassed about my body.	I don't have to deal with my feelings about my body if I stay home.	My friends think I don't like them and have stopped calling. I feel lonely.

What discoveries did you make by filling out the chart?

_____

_____

_____

_____

activity 60 ✱ showing yourself compassion, once again

for you to know

If you found that on balance, making your body your fortress is taking more away than it's giving you, you may be ready to begin making peace with your body so you can start living a more fulfilling life. The first step is showing compassion for your fears and anxieties. Self-compassion is essential in helping you move out of this fortress and into the world.

for you to do

How much compassion are you feeling right now for the ways you have protected yourself by using your body as your fortress? Write some compassionate statements below. For example:

I've always felt insecure, so I've protected myself from possible rejection by blaming my insecurities on my body. This has kept me from improving other parts of myself, like studying more to feel smarter, or taking the risk to talk to people, so I don't feel like such an outcast. I've been so scared to face my issues! Wow, how clever I've been to find this way to protect myself, when I didn't know what else to do.

Your turn:

_____

_____

_____

_____

_____

_____

_____

_____

_____

_____

If you're still having problems unlocking the key to your fortress, it might be helpful to talk with a counselor to get some support in helping you through this.

activity 61 ✳ rejecting the foe

for you to know

Not only can negative feelings about your body keep you from experiencing life, they can also turn your body into your foe. As a result, you may be spending many hours feeling bad about yourself.

for you to do

Over the course of a day, from eight a.m. to eight p.m., mark how many negative thoughts you have about your body in each hour.

Hour	Number of negative body thoughts
8:00 a.m.	
9:00 a.m.	
10:00 a.m.	
11:00 a.m.	
12:00 p.m.	
1:00 p.m.	

2:00 p.m.	
3:00 p.m.	
4:00 p.m.	
5:00 p.m.	
6:00 p.m.	
7:00 p.m.	
8:00 p.m.	

Were you surprised by the number of negative body thoughts you had? _____

How do you think these negative thoughts affect how you feel about life?

_____

_____

_____

_____

What are some ways your life might improve if you could wipe out these negative thoughts? For example, you might make room to think about sports or friends or fun activities.

_____

_____

_____

_____

_____

_____

_____

activity 62 ✳ making your body your temple

for you to know

A temple is sacred and special. It's often a place of devotion, where you can show respect and honor what's important to you. If you've found that making your body your fortress or your foe has kept you from enjoying life, then it's time to learn ways to make your body your temple.

Here are some ways you can show respect to your body:

- Accept that all bodies come in different sizes and shapes, including yours.

- Recognize the many miraculous things your body can do.

- Feel grateful for your body's abilities.

- Take care of your body's needs.

- Honor your hunger and fullness.

- Say nice things about your body.

- Wear comfortable clothes that you enjoy.

- Do nurturing things for your body.

- Stop comparing your body to others.

for you to do

Pick three of the suggestions above, and consider how you can practice them in your life. For example, if you decide to spend more time feeling grateful for your body's abilities, you could take a moment after playing a sport to reflect on your gratitude for how your body moved and how good it felt to be active.

First suggestion: _____

_____

_____

_____

Second suggestion: _____

_____

_____

_____

Third suggestion: _____

_____

_____

_____

Where will you start?

_____

_____

Eventually, you can practice all of these ways. Start slowly and build your list of the ways you show your body respect.

activity 63 ✳ accepting mother nature's plan

for you to know

Have you ever tried to make your size eight foot fit into a friend's size five shoe? Tried to get taller by stretching as far as you can every day? Used eye drops to try to change the color of your eyes? You probably haven't done any of these things, because you realize how ridiculous they are. You accept that your foot can't get smaller or that your height is (or will end up being) what Mother Nature programmed for you. You know that eye drops will never turn your brown eyes blue. But so many teens (and adults) think they can change their size or shape by going on diets or overexercising. The truth is that weight and shape are programmed by your genetics, the same way that foot size, height, and eye color are.

You learned about the dangers of dieting in Chapter 1. So if you can't really change your weight or shape because you've inherited them, the best and healthiest thing you can do is to accept in every cell of your body what Mother Nature intended for you. It takes a lot of courage to do this, but it will save you the agony of your failed attempts!

for you to do

Are you feeling even the tiniest amount of relief when you think about letting go of the fantasy of changing your body? Maybe you're feeling angry that you can't do this, or maybe you're in a little denial, because you've read about actors who've done it, so why not you? (Fact: Even people you think look amazing and perfect can't change things they dislike about their bodies. Instead, photographers have ways to digitally alter the size of their bodies, or film them in a certain light to look thinner or hide cellulite or blemishes. And for those who restrict their food or overexercise to lose weight or bulk up their muscles, the results are only temporary and possibly dangerous.)

In the lines below, write your feelings about accepting Mother Nature's plan for the aspects of your body you've wished you could change. Name those aspects and what you can do to help make acceptance more possible.

For example, when Molly saw that her life was no better after losing weight (and, of course, gaining it back), she decided to feel grateful for the body she has and began to focus on the many ways she could feel better. She started taking her piano practices seriously and became proud of the music she played.

_____

_____

_____

_____

_____

_____

_____

You can absolutely make your body feel the best it can by moving it regularly and giving it the fuel it needs each day. You can feel stronger, have more stamina and energy, and feel more physically capable—that's for sure.

In the lines below, write about the ways you could (and already do!) help your whole body feel better physically. For example:

- You could spend a few minutes stretching each day to keep your muscles limber.

- You could make sure to include some calcium-rich foods each day to strengthen your bones (more on that in the last chapter).

- You could eat enough food each day to meet your energy needs, so you can accomplish all your tasks.

- You could commit to regularly practicing your sport, dance, or gymnastics to be on top of your game.

_____

_____

_____

_____

_____

activity 64 ✳ recognizing the many miraculous things your body can do

for you to know

Since there's no healthy way to change your size or shape, you'll feel better if you focus on all the amazing things your body can do. There are so many, and they're happening all the time, from your heart beating nonstop for *decades* to hearing a bird sing or a wave crash to rolling down a grassy hill.

for you to do

Molly identified some of the amazing things her body can do:

being a good dancer

being a good hugger

taking a walk along the beach barefoot

helping Grandma carry heavy things

flying a kite

playing with Clara **(her little sister).**

throwing balls for Toffee **(her dog)** in the backyard

Name some amazing things your body can do.

_____

_____

_____

_____

_____

_____

activity 65 ✳ finding even more gratitude

for you to know

Now that you've spent some time appreciating what your body can do, focusing on gratitude will remind you to think positively about your body. Maybe you're grateful for the home run you hit or for how good it feels to slather on lotion.

for you to do

Start each morning with a body gratitude list. Practice making your first gratitude list here, and continue this regularly in your notebook. The first line is something Molly is grateful for.

I am grateful for:
The fact that I have rhythm and love to dance.

activity 66 ✳ taking care of your body's needs

for you to know

Self-care plays just as big a part in showing self-respect as it does in helping you cope with your emotions. The most basic way to show respect to the temple that is your body is to practice some of the self-care habits you worked on in the last chapter; for example, cleanliness, nourishment, sleep, and movement. Eating when you're moderately hungry and stopping when you're comfortably full are also signs of loving and respectful self-care.

for you to do

Look back at activity 50. In what ways has your self-care changed since you committed to improving it? For example, if you have focused on getting more sleep or are less sedentary, do you find that you feel better physically?

List the ways you're taking better care of your body:

_____

_____

_____

_____

_____

Write about any ideas or plans you have for improving your self-care in ways that are specifically about honoring the temple that is your body.

_____

_____

_____

_____

activity 67 ✳ saying nice things about your body

for you to know

If you take a few moments to listen to some of the ways your friends talk about their bodies, you'll probably notice that there's a lot of negative self-talk filling the air. You may also be contributing to this toxic air. These body-bashing comments can sting and make you and others feel really bad.

for you to do

Pay attention to body talk in your group of friends for a few days. When friends are changing for PE or a sport, do they look in the mirror and make negative comments? When you go shopping, are you hearing disrespectful messages about their bodies? Or if you're looking at a magazine, or watching a TV show or movie with friends, do they put themselves down, while looking at images of celebrities?

Put a check next to any negative comments you've heard from others or made about yourself. Then add any others:

Negative comment	Heard from someone else	Said it yourself
"I'm too big."		
"I hate my body."		
"My arms aren't muscular enough."		
"My stomach isn't flat enough."		
"I'm too short."		
"I don't feel pretty (or handsome)."		
"My waist is too big."		
"I'm too skinny."		
"I'm too tall."		

Find a way to change each comment to one that is positive and self-respectful. For example:

Negative comment—"I'm too big."

Positive change—"My body is curvy, just like my mom's and just like Mother Nature meant it to be."

Negative comment—"My arms aren't muscular enough."

Positive change—"I'm actually pretty strong, so I guess my muscles work when they need to."

Change some of your own negative comments to positive ones:

Negative comment: _____

Positive change: _____

Negative comment: _____

Positive change: _____

Negative comment: _____

Positive change: _____

activity 68 ✳ wearing comfortable clothes you enjoy

for you to know

Keeping clothes in your closet that fit you when you were younger or when you dieted (before the diet failed) is a surefire way to make you feel miserable. If you try to wear these clothes, they're tight and binding. If you can't even get them on, you may feel frustrated and angry. The truth is that these clothes are not meant to fit your "here and now" body. You've either outgrown them, or they are simply clothes that were meant for someone whose size or shape is different from yours.

for you to do

Here are some steps to help you become more comfortable in your clothes:

- Box up all the clothes in your closet that don't properly fit you.

- Also box up the clothes that don't give you any joy when you wear them.

- Find a charity that will be happy to take these clothes. (If you're not ready to give away the boxes, store them until you are.)

- Try on your underwear, and get rid of what isn't comfortable.

- When you can afford it, buy a few new outfits that fit comfortably and put a smile on your face.

If you followed any of these steps, how did it feel to let go of these uncomfortable clothes? It's possible you'll feel freer and more respectful toward your body. Write about your feelings here, whatever they are:

_____

_____

_____

_____

activity 69 ✳ doing nurturing things for your body

for you to know

If you have a car, have you ever spent time washing and polishing it? I'll bet it makes you happy to look at your clean and shiny baby! Or do you have some leather boots or a good leather purse? If you've rubbed conditioner into them, they're probably smoother to the touch. And do you ever pet or brush your dog or cat? They definitely love it! But what about your body?

In the last chapter, you practiced nurturing your emotions. Some of the same things are good for loving and caring for your body:

- Wear aftershave or cologne to smell nice.

- Ask someone to give you a massage. (If you can afford it, a professional massage is a great stress reducer.)

- Get a manicure or pedicure.

- Soak your skin in lotion.

- Get enough sleep. (There's that sleep thing again!)

- Get as many hugs as you can from people you love.

- Take a bubble bath or a hot shower.

- Walk barefoot in the grass.

- Dangle your feet in a swimming pool, or slide in and swim for fun.

- If you belong to a gym, sit in the steam room or sauna.

- Put a yoga or meditation app on your phone, and practice a few minutes a day.

- Do some deep breathing when you're feeling tense.

for you to do

One of the most satisfying ways to show respect to your body is to nurture it every way you can. List three body-nurturing things (from the list above or anything else you can think of) you can do this week:

1. _____

2. _____

3. _____

At the end of the week, write about how you felt afterward. Did you feel calmer, more satisfied, soothed, or anything else?

_____

_____

_____

_____

activity 70 ✳ stopping comparisons

for you to know

The clearest sign of body acceptance and respect is when you stop checking out others' bodies to see how you match up. Comparing yourself to others can only make you feel envious and dislike yourself more, or make you feel superior if you think your body is better. Neither of these feelings is comfortable, and both can cause you a great deal of pain. Envy means you're focusing on what you don't have, and superiority is shallow and short-lived.

The best thing you can do is to forget about others—your own personal qualities are what counts!

for you to do

Check all the personal qualities you possess:

☐ sense of humor ☐ generosity

☐ kindness ☐ loving-kindness

☐ self-compassion ☐ empathy

☐ commitment ☐ ability to listen

☐ work ethic ☐ loyalty

☐ dependability ☐ compassion

☐ patience ☐ honesty

☐ intelligence ☐ reliability

☐ personality ☐ courage to speak up

☐ friendship ☐ resilience

☐ talent ☐ authenticity

☐ other: _____

☐ other: _____

☐ other: _____

Now, think of someone you admire. Go back to the list and put a check next to the qualities you see in that person.

If you didn't add the person's size or shape, your authentic self (the inner part of you that holds your wisdom about who you really are) knows that the qualities on the list are what make that person (and you) special—not how someone looks!

more to do

Notice when you begin to compare yourself to another this week. As soon as you do, remember your list of personal qualities. Write about how it feels to honor yourself rather than envying others:

_____

_____

_____

_____

_____

even more to do

And here's another way to stop comparing—throw out your scale! When you weigh yourself regularly, you're actually comparing your weight that day with your weight from another day (or to some friend's or celebrity's weight.) You learned in Chapter 1 that weighing gives power to the scale instead of your inner wisdom about eating. It can also affect your feelings, as the number goes up or down.

After throwing out your scale, what feelings came up for you, either positive or negative, or both?

_____

_____

_____

_____

_____

activity 71 ✱ changing your social media habits

for you to know

One of the most effective ways to help you stop comparing is to notice just how powerful social media can be in making you feel "less than." The effortless-looking, perfect selfies may have taken the poster hours of planning and editing to achieve, and they can make you feel terrible by comparison in seconds flat.

for you to do

How often do you see pictures in your feed of people promoting their own "perfect" bodies? How does that make you feel?

_____

_____

_____

How much work do you think went into making one of these posts? What do you think the posters get out of obsessing over their social media images?

_____

_____

As your first step in letting go of social media that makes you feel bad, commit to unfollowing and unsubscribing anyone who posts these pictures or talks about dieting or unrealistic body goals. Your next step: find people who have body-positive thinking and intentions. And if you can follow people who promote intuitive eating, all the better!

Name the accounts you've deleted:

_____

_____

_____

Now name the positive ones you've added:

_____

_____

_____

After a week of making these changes, how do you feel?

_____

_____

_____

_____

_____

_____

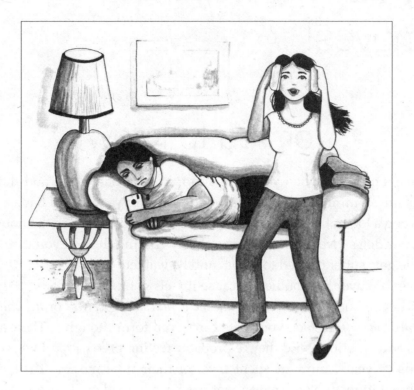

chapter 9

Joyful Movement

Luke is a teen I've known since he was very young. He told me, "My mom has been after me all my life to get off the couch and exercise. The more she pushed and cajoled me, the deeper I dug into the couch, watching more and more TV, playing more video games, and eventually adding social media to the mix. I refused and rebelled because I thought she wanted me to exercise so I'd lose weight, and because I thought of exercise as a chore. I wonder if there's another way to think about it."

The next Intuitive Eating principle is called Exercise—Feel the Difference. But since I mix things up a lot, how about using the word "movement" when you think about moving your body, instead of "exercise"? In this chapter, you'll learn why I like the idea of movement better than exercise, what the acronym NEAT means, why you might resist "exercise," and why it's important to find ways to include joyful movement into your life.

activity 72 ✳ every living thing moves!

for you to know

Did you ever have a goldfish when you were a kid? You probably did, and did you notice that that fish spent its life swimming around the bowl? Or better yet, do you have a cat or dog? Your cat may love to sleep a lot, but when she's up, she chases dust bunnies in the house or birds in the backyard. And your dog's favorite activity is probably chasing the ball you throw, and when you jingle his leash, he gets super excited to go out and be walked.

Your pets love to move their bodies, because it feels good, and because they have an innate desire to move. They're not thinking *If I run in the yard, I'll lose weight*, or *If I build my muscles, the other dogs will think I'm buff*. In fact, your pets can't even form thoughts. Their actions are based on their instincts and emotions, and they're probably feeling pretty joyful when they're moving.

For thousands of years, humans spent most of their time moving their bodies, but more recently, with a burst in technology, movement has been turned on its head. People spend many hours in front of TVs or computers, attached to their phones, or simply lying around.

for you to do

During the next week, pay attention to the ways that animals and people move—not how they exercise, but just how they move. For example, you might see your cat stretching her paws or kids running around a playground. List all the activities you notice:

_____

_____

_____

_____

_____

Write about your observations of all this movement. For example, did it seem forced or natural? Did you notice some people or pets moving around a lot and others barely moving?

_____

_____

_____

_____

_____

_____

activity 73 ✳ exploring exercise vs. movement

for you to know

At the movies in the mall, I've noticed that most people take the escalator, rather than walking up the stairs. No matter how crowded the escalator, people just avoid the stairs. I see this happening in lots of other places too. I don't think people do this because they're necessarily lazy. Instead, I think it's probably because many people have black-and-white ideas about exercise. To them, exercise means working out at the gym or running a few miles on the street. If they've already exercised that day, they think, *Why bother walking upstairs?* The rest of the time, they can justify being sedentary. And others don't even think about moving at all!

for you to do

For a week, keep track of the ways you move (both simple movement and exercise), and mark how each feels. (You might need to add two checks for some.) The first couple of rows were how Luke began his chart.

Activity	Pleasant (pleasurable, enjoyable, fun, joyful)	Unpleasant (distasteful, difficult, uncomfortable)
Played basketball with my brother	√	
Hiked with my mom		√

Look over your list of physical activities, and write about your relationship with movement. For example, are some of the ways you move your body pleasurable and joyful for you, or do you find them uncomfortable, or even miserable? Which activities feel the best for you?

_____

_____

_____

_____

_____

_____

more to do

Evaluate whether you're primarily an exerciser or a mover:

1. Do you think you're exercising only if you're at the gym, using exercise equipment?

2. Do you park a distance from your destination so you can get some walking in?

3. On a day you've worked out, do you think it's okay to spend the rest of the day lying on your bed or couch?

4. Would you rather work out at the gym than just be active?

5. Do you take the stairs instead of the escalator if they're available?

6. If you have a two-story house, when you forget something upstairs, do you see it as an opportunity for movement?

If you answered yes to questions 1, 3, and 4, you're likely an exerciser.
If you answered yes to questions 2, 5, and 6, you're likely a mover.
(Or, maybe, movement isn't a big part of your life at all.)

If you found that you're mostly an exerciser, write about whether you're willing to also become a mover. By the way, if you do love to exercise or work out, that's cool—don't give it up! Just think about adding other everyday movement into your life, as well. Read on for why!

_____

_____

_____

_____

_____

_____

_____

_____

activity 74 ✳ learning about NEAT

for you to know

Are you thinking, *Is she telling me that I need to clean up my room?* Nope, I'm not your parent, although cleaning up your room is definitely an activity that keeps you moving! NEAT is an acronym for **non-exercise activity thermogenesis**. It basically means that your body is creating heat by simply moving around. NEAT happens when you're not sleeping or eating and doesn't include formal exercise. Here are some NEAT activities:

wiggling your toes

standing up

walking up stairs

walking on level ground

playing with your dog

washing a car

pacing around the room

standing on one leg

dancing

Are you getting the idea? These NEAT activities are all examples of simply moving your body as you go through your day, in contrast to having an intense burst of exercise at the gym or running a half marathon. Interestingly, people are often healthier when they move much of the time, rather than scheduling formal exercise and then lying around for hours watching movies and checking their feeds.

Can you think of some ways to put more NEAT in your life? Some examples might be:

- Take the stairs instead of an escalator or elevator.

- Stretch your body when you get up in the morning.

- Put on some music and dance.

- Park a couple of blocks away from where you're going, so you can walk farther.

List some NEAT activities you could add into your life:

_____

_____

_____

_____

_____

activity 75 ✳ being sedentary

for you to know

Being sedentary means tending to spend much of your time sitting, being inactive, and having little physical movement. Teens are often sedentary because of technology, homework demands, and social and school commitments. And sometimes they're just rebelling from all the pressure they feel to exercise, like Luke did. In past chapters, you learned about how powerful your need to rebel can be when told what to do. In this case, the sad part about rebelling by being sedentary is that you tend to feel pretty lousy physically.

Unfortunately, being sedentary not only affects how you feel from day to day but is also associated with some health risks, like bone or muscle loss, mood swings, slowed metabolism, and possibly heart and brain problems and diabetes—things that won't affect you now, but are important to keep in mind for the future.

for you to do

For this exercise, pay attention to the amount of time you spend sitting, doing sedentary activities. Add any activities that aren't listed.

Sedentary activity	Hours during the week	Hours on the weekend
Driving		
Sitting in class		
Doing homework		
Talking on the phone		
Surfing the internet		
Checking social media		
Watching television		
Playing video games		
Reading for pleasure		
Lounging with friends		
Sitting at the movies		
Total hours per day:		

How many hours were you sedentary on weekdays? _____

On weekends? _____

Which sedentary activities do you do most often?

_____

_____

_____

more to do

In the chart below, mark any of the physical or emotional symptoms you may feel as a result of being sedentary, and add any others.

Low energy	
Achy muscles	
Tiredness	
No stamina	
Stiffness	
Weakness	
Feeling isolated from friends	
Feeling inferior to athletic or active friends	

Write about any symptoms you may have noticed by being sedentary and how this might affect the quality of your life.

_____

_____

_____

_____

At school you're probably standing up about every hour in order to go on to your next class, but you may be super sedentary on weekends and long vacations at home. What's pretty exciting is that simply standing up regularly throughout the day will keep you from being sedentary. When you're not in class, stand up for about five minutes each half hour. You can also move around and stretch during this time. Just think about how much "neater" you're becoming!

activity 76 ✳ wondering about exercise resistance

for you to know

If you discovered that you find exercise to be a drag and that your relationship with movement tends to be negative, you may have had some troublesome experiences in the past. Here are some reasons why you might resist physical activity:

- A parent has pushed you to exercise, saying that it's for your health, when you really know you're being judged for your weight and pressed to exercise to lose weight.

- Maybe you had an injury in a sport or in dance or gymnastics. While healing from the injury, you can't move your body the way you like. After the injury heals, you sometimes can't perform as well as before or are afraid you'll hurt yourself again.

- If you're forced to do the same activity your family does, and you don't really like it, you can end up resenting movement and rebelling against it.

- If you've bought into the culturally thin or muscular ideal, and you don't feel that your body matches up to that ideal, it's possible that you shun movement because you don't want others to judge your body.

- If exercise has always been connected with dieting, which has felt like a failure, it's possible that you've thrown out movement along with the failed diet.

- If you can't meet an unrealistic goal, you figure, *Why bother!*

for you to do

If any of these reasons for exercise resistance fits for you, write about your experience (there could be more than one):

_____

_____

_____

_____

Be compassionate toward yourself for reacting the way you have. As an intuitive eater, you learn to listen to your body's signals, rather than reacting to external issues. You've rejected movement as a way to protect you from the feelings that may have come up in these situations. Now is the time to heal your resistance by paying attention to how great movement can make your body feel.

activity 77 ✳ why include movement?

for you to know

Now that you've had a chance to think about whether and why you may resist exercise and how that feels, or whether you've been sedentary as a habit, let's look at the reasons to include movement in your life and how you might do that.

Here are some things that being active and moving your body can do for you:

make you stronger

give you more energy

increase balance

increase stamina

help you sleep better

make you feel less tired during the day

keep you from getting sick

keep your heart healthy

strengthen your bones

reduce stress

improve mood

increase alertness

improve learning and memory

increase metabolism

help you identify hunger and fullness signals

give you joy

The bottom line is that if you become more active and include more movement in your life, your mind and body will feel so much better!

for you to do

Close your eyes, and imagine how your life might improve if you got some of the benefits of movement listed above. Write down what you've imagined:

_____

_____

_____

_____

_____

_____

_____

more to do

Here's a list of activities that some teens do. Mark the ones you do now and whether they bring you joy. Add any others that you enjoy. Then mark the ones you'd like to include in your life:

Activity	Do now	Brings you joy	Might like to do
Walking			
Running			
Hiking			
Biking			
Swimming			
Dancing			
Basketball			
Baseball			
Football			
Volleyball			
Hockey			
Archery			
Surfing			
Boogie boarding			
Skiing (downhill or cross country)			
Snowboarding			
Roller skating			

Roller blading			
Skateboarding			
Ice-skating			
Martial arts			
Pilates			
Gyrotonics			
Yoga			
Ping-Pong			
Tennis			
Paintballing			
Rock climbing			
Trampoline			
Boxing			
Weight lifting			
Playing with your dog			
Jumping rope			
Aerobics			
Bowling			

Some people like to exercise. Others don't. But if you can find an activity that brings you joyful movement and keeps you from being sedentary, you will become a healthier, active person who feels better physically and emotionally. You'll probably get sick less often, have more energy, sleep better, and be able to concentrate better at school.

even more to do

List three activities you put in the "might like to do" column above, and plan when you could put them in your schedule. After you've done each of the activities, notice how it felt physically and emotionally to be active.

Activity you'll do	When will you do it?	How did you feel afterward?

activity 78 ✳ recognizing overexercising

for you to know

We've spent a lot of time talking about the benefits of movement and finding movement that feels joyous to you. You've learned that you don't have to do structured exercise to be healthy. We've also looked at the problems with being sedentary. But what about the opposite? What happens when you move too much?

Here are some reasons why people overexercise:

- They worry that if they don't exercise enough, they'll gain weight.

- They think it's healthier if they do excessive amounts of exercise.

- They feel bad about themselves if they're not pushing themselves.

- They think that just moving around isn't enough.

These people will exercise even if they're sick, overtired, or don't really have time on a particular day. They turn exercise into a chore, rather than a joy. But overexercising can

cause you to burn out and end up becoming sedentary;

cause injury;

be used as a way of escaping feelings;

raise your risk of getting sick;

keep you from doing other important things in your life;

slow your metabolism, if you're not eating enough.

for you to do

So how do you find the right amount of movement for you? Here are some questions to ask to get the right answer:

- Does the movement I do make me feel good?

- Does it make me angry or resentful?

- Does it often cause me to get injured, overtired, or sick?

- Does it give me joy?

- Can I fit it into my life and still keep up my homework, social and family life, and fun times?

Let's be real. As a teen, you're being stretched in so many ways. You may often feel overwhelmed trying to get everything done. If your need to move feels compulsive and makes it difficult to live a balanced life, then it's too much. If the amount you move causes injuries, being sick a lot, or feeling exhausted, then it's too much. The right amount of movement will be different for each person. If movement gives you joy and makes you feel healthier and stronger, and you're able to include it with the other important things in your life, then you're doing just the right amount. And remember, movement doesn't necessarily mean formal exercise. Being active and including NEAT in your life on a daily basis will make you healthy, happy, and fit!

After answering all of the questions above, evaluate the amount of movement in your life, and decide whether it's not enough, too much, or just right.

_____

_____

_____

_____

_____

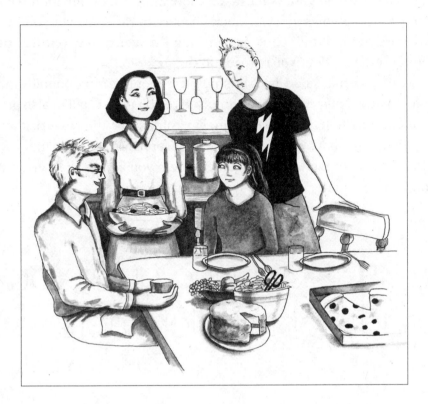

chapter 10

From Nutrition to Play Food—
Room for It All

Olivia is a teen whose parents love her very much and want her to have the best in life. Olivia told me, "My mom has been cooking for me all my life. She's a great cook, but she's always trying to control what I eat. She only wants me to eat 'healthy' food. When she sees me eating chips or dessert at our cousins' house, she gives me the evil eye. It's always made me feel so guilty. Couldn't I be healthy and still eat chips and cookies? I'm so sick of feeling guilty!"

The last principle of Intuitive Eating is Honor Your Health with Gentle Nutrition. Putting nutrition at the end was very purposeful, and even though I've presented some other principles out of order, I felt strongly that keeping it last in this workbook made the most sense. And here's why—if you start thinking about nutrition before you've made full peace with food or you're still having diet thoughts or you haven't figured out how to get the most satisfaction out of eating, a focus on nutrition is going to backfire on you. Wanting to know more about nutrition has to come from a very deep place in you that knows you can always choose to eat whatever you like, without judgment. When you're truly at that point and are noticing that you'd like to feel better physically or are simply curious about nutrition, you're ready to dig in.

I'm going to show you that good health is not just about getting enough nutrition but also about making room for the "play foods" that simply give you pleasure! I'm also going to teach you some basic facts about nutrition. But, once again, I'm going to be the maverick and let you know that rather than telling you what to eat, I trust that you were born with the inner wisdom to guide you about how to nourish yourself. I'm just going to help you add to that wisdom by giving you some information to help you decide the best way to eat *for you*.

activity 79 ✻ figuring out if you're really ready for nutrition facts

for you to know

Have you ever heard your mom or dad (or grandma or anyone else) say, "Finish your meal before you eat your dessert"? Or "You've had enough junk food—eat something healthy!!" If so, it's likely that you've taken in some misconceptions about the "right" way to eat or have had some negative reactions to what they say to you about nutrition.

for you to do

To figure out if you're ready to learn about nutrition, answer yes or no to these questions, and total your responses in the last line:

Question	Yes	No	Chapter
Do I truly feel I can eat anything I want without internal judgment?			3
Do I notice how my body feels based on what I choose to eat?			2, 5, 6
Do I think I could improve how I feel physically by knowing more about nutrition?			8
Do I want to learn about nutrition to be healthy in the future?			6, 7
Have I learned to eat for pleasure and satisfaction?			2
Do I have healthy coping mechanisms for my emotions?			7
Can I recognize when I'm hungry?			5
Can I recognize when I'm full?			6
Can I tolerate the sadness I feel when I stop eating because I'm full?			7
Do I respect and appreciate my body?			8
Have I let go of any ideas about dieting in order to change my body?			1
Have I incorporated movement in my life in order to feel better?			9
Am I brave enough to speak up for how and what I want to eat?			4
Am I willing to challenge food fads and the myths I hear?			1
Do I want to learn how to eat for optimal energy and well-being?			7
Have I let go of any judgment about my food or weight?			1, 3, 8
Have I let go of any judgment about others' food or weight?			1, 3, 8
Do I believe that my body knows how to guide me in my food choices?			1, 3
Totals:			

If you answered yes to at least sixteen of the questions, you're good to go for the rest of this chapter. If there are still quite a few no answers, you might want to wait to read this chapter until you've moved further along in your journey toward intuitive eating. Remember, have no judgment about your progress. This is a process that takes as long as it needs to take. You will eventually get there!

more to do

List the questions that had a no answer for you:

_____

_____

_____

_____

_____

In the right-hand column above, there is a key to the chapters you might want to reread for each of the questions.

activity 80 ✳ paying attention to how eating can affect how you feel

for you to know

Have you ever wondered why some days you feel livelier and more alert than others? If you have, it's likely that you know that getting enough sleep definitely affects how you feel. But what you eat also has a strong impact on your energy levels and physical well-being. Having a steady flow of nutrition throughout the day will keep your energy up. Learning about which foods might give your body discomfort will prevent distress and help you feel good all day.

Here are some ways eating affects how you feel, and why:

- Eating breakfast will set your hunger and fullness signals for the whole day.

- Eating about every three to four hours will keep your blood sugar even and keep you from going into primal hunger.

- Eating balanced meals that have some protein, carbohydrate, and fat will satisfy your body better than a "mono" meal (a meal with only one item).

- Eating foods with staying power (that is, foods that take longer to digest than others) will give you plenty of energy until you can eat again.

- Eating "air foods" like popcorn or Pirate's Booty fills you up fast, but you'll get hungry again very quickly.

- Speed of eating matters. Too fast can give you indigestion. Eating slowly allows your body to digest your food more efficiently.

- Certain foods can affect your stomach and cause gas or give you a stomachache. Others give you no problems.

- Eating too much food or foods that make you feel overfull can make you uncomfortable.

for you to do

For one full day, pay attention to some of the factors mentioned above, and use the chart that follows to note how you feel. If you do this exercise twice—once on a school day, and once on a weekend day—you'll get even more information about how food affects you. (You'll find a copy of this chart at http://www.newharbinger.com/41443.)

Here are some of the body feelings to consider, with some examples from Olivia's eating day in the first two lines:

felt too full

stayed full too long

didn't hold me very long—got hungry too soon

felt satisfied

stomach hurt

headache

indigestion (gas, bloating)

Time	Food(s) eaten	How you felt after eating
9:00 a.m.	Muffin and coffee	Fine, but got hungry after an hour and couldn't concentrate.
12:00 noon	Cheeseburger, fries, and onion rings	Tasted great. Ate it fast, felt too full, and got indigestion.

What did you learn about how food affects you physically?

_____

_____

_____

_____

_____

Use what you discovered in this exercise to help you make your best food choices.

activity 81 ✳ learning exactly what nutrition is

for you to know

You may hear some of these words from your parents, teachers, coaches, or doctors on a regular basis:

"Make sure you get enough nutrition."

"You haven't eaten anything nutritious all day."

"Nutrition is the key to health."

Any idea what nutrition actually means? It's all about the chemicals in foods that nourish and give energy to your body and your mind, help you grow and be strong, and keep you healthy.

So, in case the idea of nutrition is a bit fuzzy, I thought I'd give you some basics. Here are some important words in the world of nutrition and what they mean:

- *Nutrients* are substances in food that are necessary for life.

- *Macronutrients* are nutrients needed in large amounts for your body to grow, function, and have energy. These include carbohydrates, proteins, and fats.

- *Carbohydrate*s are substances you need in the largest amount, as the body's main source of fuel to create energy. If you don't get enough carbohydrates, you'll burn proteins and fats as fuel, which will keep them from being available for the jobs they must do.

  Important note: We seem to be living in a world these days that is "carb-phobic." You may be getting lots of messages from friends or media that try to make you afraid of eating carbohydrates. But here's an interesting fact—the only energy source that can get into your brain is glucose, which comes from the breakdown of carbohydrates. And the brain uses about a fifth of your total calories a day—all from carbohydrates! (And just so you know, the word "calorie" means a unit or measure of heat energy.) If you don't get enough carbs, you'll release NPY (remember, from the hunger chapter?), which will send you out on a quest to get as many carbs as you can find!

- *Fiber* is a form of carbohydrate that the body can't digest but that is needed to make your gastrointestinal tract work properly and help you notice fullness.

- *Protein* makes up most cells and organs of the body. It's necessary for growth, strong muscles, healthy hair and nails, repairing tissues, and making hormones that regulate the body and enzymes that are needed for all biochemical reactions in the body.

- *Fat*s (also called lipids) don't dissolve in water and are needed to make cell membranes and some vitamins, carry fat-soluble vitamins into the body, make receptors for brain chemicals, protect inner organs, and keep you warm. Fat molecules also hold the flavor in foods and keep you satisfied longer.

- *Micronutrients* are chemicals needed in tiny amounts that include *vitamins* and *minerals*, used to maintain health; regulate your heart and the rest of your body; help you grow and have strong bones (calcium and vitamins D and K are especially important for your bones); help prevent disease; and help your blood clot, your muscles contract, and your nervous system function.

At http://www.newharbinger.com/41443, you'll find a chart of macro- and micronutrients, with some examples of foods where you can find them.

for you to do

Olivia used a similar chart as before, but instead of writing about how she felt after she ate, she wrote down some of the nutrients in the foods she ate. You can use the chart to note the nutrients in your foods. (You'll find a copy of this chart at http://www.newharbinger.com/41443.)

Time	Food(s) eaten	Nutrients
9:00 a.m.	Muffin and coffee	Carbohydrates, fat
12:00 noon	Cheeseburger, fries, and onion rings	Protein, carbohydrates, fat, fiber, vitamins, and minerals

Look over your chart to see if any nutrients are missing or only in short supply. For example, was there a lot of carbohydrate but not much fiber? Was there a lot of fat but not much protein? Were there very few sources of vitamins and minerals?

_____

_____

_____

_____

more to do

Write down any changes you might want to make in your eating to fill in some of the nutrients that were low or missing. For example, you might want to include more fruits and vegetables that will give you more vitamins, minerals, and fiber, or you might want to add more foods high in protein.

_____

_____

_____

_____

activity 82 ✱ exploring how play food fits in

for you to know

Adequate nutrition may be about your physical health, but your emotional health is equally important. As an intuitive eater, a part of your emotional health rests on feeling comfortable eating all foods, without judgment or guilt. That's where play food fits in. Play food is food that's pretty low in some of the nutrients you've learned about. It's the food that most people call junk food, but as I mentioned in an earlier chapter, I don't like to call it junk, because I truly believe it has a place in our lives. (After all, we throw junk in the trash!) The goal is to make all foods emotionally equal, even if they're not nutritionally equal. Sure, some foods contain more nutrition than others, but you want to have the same positive feelings about eating apple pie as you do apples. This is where your inner intuitive wisdom comes in. With the freedom to eat whatever you like any time you like, eventually you're going to get a pretty good balance of very nutritious food, with some play food along the way, just like those toddlers I told you about earlier.

for you to do

To help you understand what I mean, I'm going to pose a couple of questions for you to think about:

1. What would your life be like if you went to school all day, every day? No weekends or holidays off? No time for being social or having fun?

   My hunch is that you let out a few big groans and thought that, although you might get super smart with all this schooling, you'd also be exhausted, frustrated, and craving time off.

2. What would your life be like if you never went to school another day in your life? Had all the time in the world to hang with your friends, doing a lot of nothing?

Here's my second hunch—after the first few yelps of joy, you'd start thinking about how little you'd learn, how hard it would be to get a job, and how bored you'd eventually get. Yes, bored! Remember the whole idea of habituation from the chapter on making peace with food? After you get the same thing over and over, its excitement level just vanishes.

Hope you're catching the metaphor and getting the idea about how play food can fit in your life. Just like you wouldn't want to be forbidden from eating it, you also naturally wouldn't want it all the time.

more to do

Pick one play food, like cookies, chips, fries, or candy. Now plan to have some of it at every meal for a whole week. Observe how many meals or days go by until you barely care about this food.

Write about your experience below:

_____

_____

_____

_____

_____

_____

activity 83 ✳ learning about commonsense nutrition

for you to know

To round out this chapter on nutrition, here are a few basic guidelines that will ensure you get all the nutrients you need in a week. I like to use a week rather than a day because I trust that your body will get plenty of what it needs throughout the week to be healthy. You don't have to get it all in one day!

- *Eat a variety of foods.* Your best bet of getting all those carbs, protein, fat, fiber, vitamins, and minerals is by mixing up your foods, not eating the same thing over and over. Every food has a different mix of nutrients—so go for variety.

- *Eat enough food* to take care of your hunger and fullness *but not so much* that you feel uncomfortably full. Remember, your body is very wise. If you eat according to hunger and fullness, you'll get plenty of nutrition without overloading your body.

- *Balance your meals, for the most part.* Just like getting a variety of foods throughout the week, eating meals that have a balance of nutrients will give you more satisfaction, make you feel better physically, and make it easier for you to get all those nutrients you need.

- *Don't get caught up in food fads and myths.* As a nutritionist for many years, I've seen ideas come and go. Whatever is seen as "bad" becomes the ideal food a few years later. It's easy to get sucked into the latest fad, cutting out certain foods, which can end up jeopardizing your overall nutrition. Just sayin'…

for you to do

To consider the value of nutrition in your life, ask yourself these questions:

Do you believe you'll be healthier and feel better if you eat foods that are nutrient-dense (contain lots of nutrients)?

_____

Do you believe your body has the wisdom to help you choose foods that will supply these nutrients?

_____

Do you feel free to eat some play food just for pleasure and know that you'll still get plenty of nutrition from other foods?

_____

Do you need more time developing your intuitive eating skills to take action on what you've learned in this chapter?

_____

Looking back at your answers, write your thoughts about how ready you feel to incorporate what you've learned about nutrition into your eating life:

_____

_____

_____

_____

_____

Finally, which information in this chapter has affected you most? And how will you include it in your life?

_____

_____

_____

_____

_____

_____

activity 84 ✳ putting it all together

for you to know

Congratulations! You have worked very hard to understand the principles of Intuitive Eating. You've learned that intuitive eating isn't just about instinct, but also includes getting comfortable with your emotions and using your rational thinking.

for you to do

This final activity will help you put everything you've learned together in one place. On the left, you'll find all the Intuitive Eating principles, with the matching chapter titles in the next column. Next to each, write some of the activities you've practiced. Finally, on a scale of 1–10, rate how well you believe you understand and are practicing the principle, and add a simple statement about where you are with it. Finally, figure out your approximate average score.

Olivia used this chart to help her come to the conclusion that she has become an intuitive eater. It helped her review the ways she used the workbook, worksheets, checklists, and journaling to help her stay on her path. You can see how she filled it out for the first two principles and what her average total score was.

Intuitive Eating principle	Chapter title	Activities practiced	How you rate (1–10)
Reject the Diet Mentality	Chapter 1: What's Wrong with Dieting?	Did History of Dieting Worksheet. Considered Pros and Cons of Dieting. Listed the tools to practice for getting rid of dieting.	10! I'll never diet again. It's not worth it!
Discover the Satisfaction Factor	Chapter 2: Savor and Be Satisfied!	Did "craving" exercise. Explored all the different mouth and body sensations. Worked on the eating environment exercises.	9. Almost there. Just need to work on not getting distracted sometimes when I'm eating.
Make Peace with Food	Chapter 3: Your License to Eat What You Like		

Challenge the Food Police	Chapter 4: Banishing the Food Police		
Honor Your Hunger	Chapter 5: Do You Hear Your Stomach Growling?		
Feel Your Fullness	Chapter 6: Full and Comfortable		
Cope with Your Emotions Without Using Food	Chapter 7: Is Food Your Frenemy?		
Respect Your Body	Chapter 8: Your Body— Temple, Fortress, or Foe?		
Exercise—Feel the Difference	Chapter 9: Joyful Movement		
Honor Your Health with Gentle Nutrition	Chapter 10: From Nutrition to Play Food— Room for It All		
Average score for all principles			9.5. I may not be perfect, but I'm an intuitive eater for the most part. That's good enough for me!

You'll find a blank chart on the next page and at http://www.newharbinger.com/41443. Use it from time to time to see the progress you're making.

Intuitive Eating principle	Chapter title	Activities practiced	How you rate (1–10)
Reject the Diet Mentality	Chapter 1: What's Wrong with Dieting?		
Discover the Satisfaction Factor	Chapter 2: Savor and Be Satisfied!		
Make Peace with Food	Chapter 3: Your License to Eat What You Like		
Challenge the Food Police	Chapter 4: Banishing the Food Police		
Honor Your Hunger	Chapter 5: Do You Hear Your Stomach Growling?		

Feel Your Fullness	Chapter 6: Full and Comfortable		
Cope with Your Emotions Without Using Food	Chapter 7: Is Food Your Frenemy?		
Respect Your Body	Chapter 8: Your Body—Temple, Fortress, or Foe?		
Exercise—Feel the Difference	Chapter 9: Joyful Movement		
Honor Your Health with Gentle Nutrition	Chapter 10: From Nutrition to Play Food—Room for It All		
Average score for all principles			

more to do

If you rated any of the principles below a 9 on the scale, you can reread their chapters and practice the activities once again. By practicing over and over, you'll find your rating improve over time. Remember, intuitive eating is about "for the most part." It's not about perfection. Progress sometimes is slow, sometimes more rapid, but eventually, you, like Olivia, will find that you feel confident in calling yourself an intuitive eater—for the most part!

Which principles and activities need more practice?

_____

_____

_____

_____

_____

_____

_____

_____

_____

_____

_____

Living the principles of Intuitive Eating will give you the freedom to trust your body to know how to eat, find great pleasure and satisfaction in eating, and develop a relationship with food and your body that is positive, life-affirming, and joyous!

Note: If you are struggling in any way and need more help than this workbook can give you, please know that it's perfectly appropriate to ask for it at any time. Here are some questions to ask yourself to see if you need to speak with a trusted adult:

- Do you feel out of control when you eat?

- Do you feel scared around food?

- Do you think about food so much that it's interfering with your life?

- Are you feeling hopeless about making changes in your eating behaviors?

- Are you having panic attacks about food or your body?

- Are you engaging in any self-harming behaviors?

- Have you been restricting amounts or types of food?

- Have you been losing weight rapidly? (Have your clothes become too loose?)

- Are you scared to ask for help?

If you answered yes to any of these questions, then these are things that are beyond the scope of this book. There is someone who can help you. A registered dietitian or nutritionist can help you with your relationship with food. A mental health professional (psychotherapist, psychiatrist, or counselor) can help you to understand and handle your emotions. You can also talk to your doctor, nurse, minister, rabbi, school counselor, or other adult you can trust.

Acknowledgments

There are a multitude of people I would like to acknowledge and thank for your inspiration, advice, support, and encouragement in making this workbook possible:

David Hale Smith, Inkwell Management, LLC, my agent, who has consistently seen the value of Intuitive Eating.

Ryan Buresh, my acquisitions editor, for your dedication to the Intuitive Eating workbooks and your desire to bring the message of Intuitive Eating to the teen world. Your responsiveness and support have meant the world to me.

Clancy Drake, my editor and editorial manager, for your guidance and input throughout the writing of this book.

Karen Schader, my copy editor, for all your compassionate help in polishing my words.

Evelyn Tribole, MS, RDN, for being my partner in the revolution that Intuitive Eating has become.

Tracy Tylka, PhD, for championing significant research validating Intuitive Eating.

Russelle Westbrook, for your unending effort in creating the "right" illustrations for this workbook.

Arlene Drake, PhD, MFT for your unselfish understanding, support, encouragement, and love throughout the writing of this book.

Karen Freeman, MS, RDN, CSSD, my dearest friend, for a lifetime of support.

Shazi Shabatian, MS, RDN, my associate, for your patience, empathy, and advice.

All the members of the professional group I supervise, as well as my professional community who are true believers in Intuitive Eating, and all my clients—teens, kids and adults—for your encouragement and excitement about this workbook.

Sumner Brooks, MPH, RDN, CEDRD, founder and producer of the EDRD Pro community; Linda Bacon, PhD, and the Health at Every Size community; Certified Intuitive Eating Counselors and Lay Facilitators; and the Intuitive Eating Online Community, for supporting and advocating Intuitive Eating.

My family and dear friends for your patience, caring, and understanding of my limited free time.

Ellen Ledley, LCSW, my therapist, for keeping me sane throughout the writing of this book.

Bonnie Kalisher, my assistant, for keeping my office running smoothly and Garry Margolis, my computer consultant, for rescuing me when my computer skills needed a boost.

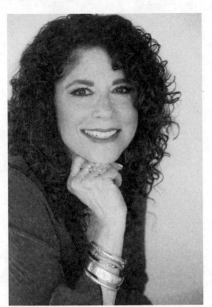

Photo by Mikel Healey

Elyse Resch, MS, RDN, CEDRD, is a nutrition therapist in private practice in Beverly Hills, CA, with over thirty-six years of experience specializing in eating disorders, intuitive eating, and health at every size. She is coauthor of *Intuitive Eating* and *The Intuitive Eating Workbook*, author of *The Intuitive Eating Workbook for Teens*, and has published journal articles, print articles, and blog posts. She also does regular speaking engagements, podcasts, and extensive media interviews. Her work has been profiled on CNN, KABC, NBC, KTTV, AP Press, KFI Radio, *USA Today*, and *The Huffington Post*, among others. Resch is nationally known for her work in helping patients break free from the diet mentality through the intuitive eating process. Her philosophy embraces the goal of developing body positivity and reconnecting with one's internal wisdom about eating. She supervises and trains health professionals, is a certified eating disorder registered dietitian, a fellow of the International Association of Eating Disorder Professionals, and a fellow of the Academy of Nutrition and Dietetics.

More 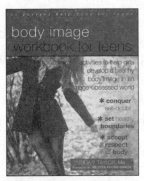 Instant Help Books for Teens

An Imprint of New Harbinger Publications

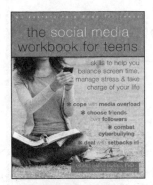
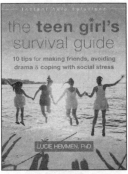
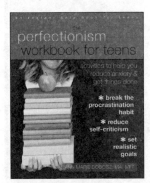
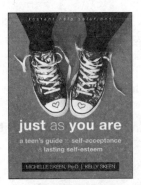
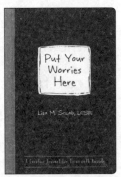 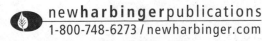

Register your **new harbinger** titles for additional benefits!

When you register your **new harbinger** title—purchased in any format, from any source—you get access to benefits like the following:

- Downloadable accessories like printable worksheets and extra content

- Instructional videos and audio files

- Information about updates, corrections, and new editions

Not every title has accessories, but we're adding new material all the time.

Access free accessories in 3 easy steps:

1. Sign in at NewHarbinger.com (or **register** to create an account).

2. Click on **register a book**. Search for your title and click the **register** button when it appears.

3. Click on the **book cover or title** to go to its details page. Click on **accessories** to view and access files.

That's all there is to it!

If you need help, visit:

NewHarbinger.com/accessories

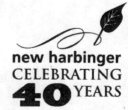

new harbinger
CELEBRATING
40 YEARS